PRAISE FOR DEMENTIA MAN

This book is a captivating and thoughtfully written account of the author's fascinating life, including the years he's spent living with dementia. Mr. Simon skillfully and vividly describes his experiences in a way that enhances the reader's understanding of what it is like for him to be living with the condition. He rightfully advocates for a world where those living with brain changes are provided adequate support, and healthcare providers offer resources instead of simply a diagnosis.

> **Teepa Snow, MS, OTR/L, FAOTA,**
> founder of Positive Approach to Care®

Samuel Simon is our fabulous teacher of how people with dementia like himself have so very much to offer us all. Sam is the Dementia Man he writes about. His performances have thrilled our medical students here at Stony Brook University, in the world of New York City theater, and all across America. His writing is so elegant that words leap off the page into mind and heart. He is a gift to us all as we seek more space and place for people with memory challenges in our lives.

Stephen G. Post, PhD,
director, Center for Medical Humanities,
Compassionate Care & Bioethics,
Stony Brook University School of Medicine

I love this book, and I love *Dementia Man*, Sam's wonderful play that has inspired so many with its honesty, passion and humor. I am deeply touched by the enthusiasm with which audience members are invited to be part of a conversation that impacts so meaningfully on their lives. I also, and perhaps especially, admire Sam for continuing to give and to perform after it became clear he needed to be holding the script—and relying on his wife, Susan, to do so. For me, this is just one of many ways Sam continues to live as a maker of "good trouble" and the commitment he and Susan have, as partners, as a family, as people of faith and members of the human community, to take all that life has thrown at them and move forward in the most giving, caring and compassionate ways possible. What a gift!

Mary Fridley,
president, Mary Fridley Associates; faculty, East Side Institute; founder, The Joy of Dementia (You Gotta Be Kidding!); and coordinator, Reimagining Dementia: A Creative Coalition for Social Justice

Sam Simon's engaging memoir offers keen insights into one man's journey with a difficult diagnosis, first of mild cognitive impairment and then with early-stage Alzheimer's disease. Too often, the voices of people living with dementia go unheard, and Mr. Simon seeks to change that, first with his play, and now in this book, bringing the rest of us into his world, where he finds meaning and purpose in his full-throated declaration, "I choose life."

George Worthington,
convenor, Dementia Friendly Central Virginia

Samuel Simon, author of the acclaimed play *Dementia Man*, has now penned a chronicle of his journey into mild cognitive impairment, followed by a diagnosis of early Alzheimer's disease. Largely autobiographical, the book (with the same title) provides rare and valuable insights into the thoughts and feelings of an affected individual as he and his caregiver/family navigate the complex and confusing health care system in the US.

As is typical of this disease, Sam's initial symptoms were brushed off as normal aging, stress, overwork, or some other etiology – leading to delays in diagnosis (averaging 2+ years). Persistence with second and third opinions finally led to an accurate diagnosis, treatment, prognosis, and opportunities to participate in clinical research.

Sam hits the nail on the head when he notes that our health care system is grossly inadequate and unprepared to care for the "silver tsunami" - the growing number of individuals affected by cognitive impairment with aging. This was only further amplified when two new treatments for those with early Alzheimer's disease – slowing the rate of cognitive and functional decline by about 30-40% - became available in 2023 and 2024. The system is now truly overwhelmed.

Sam also notes the lack of societal accommodations for those with cognitive impairment, while individuals with physical challenges benefit from now routine adaptations including wheelchair ramps, braille elevator buttons, and talking or chirping signals at crosswalks. Ever "the troublemaker" (self-described), he ends with a list of societal adaptations (demands?) to assist those with cognitive impairments, including the assignment of a navigator for much-needed education and guidance.

I also agree with Sam that the word *dementia* may be degrading and insulting to some, and therefore should be retired (as we have already discarded *retarded*, *Mongoloid*, and many other labels). So, I have tried to not use it here.

This book will be appreciated by the millions of older individuals who may recognize all-too-familiar symptoms in themselves, as well as a helpful guide to family members and clinicians who wish to better understand those affected by this devastating disorder. A list of helpful organizations and websites will also be appreciated by many who may find themselves in similar circumstances—if not now, maybe later.

R. Scott Turner, PhD, MD,
professor of neurology, MedStar Georgetown University Hospital, Washington, DC
director, Memory Disorders Program, Georgetown University

Since beginning our work together on the stage play of *Dementia Man* as part of the 2023 Dementia Arts Fellowship, Sam Simon has exhibited the type of good trouble every health care practitioner appreciates. He is tireless in his advocating for better treatment, equitable access to care, and the dignity so often stripped from those living with dementia, Alzheimer's disease, and other cognitive impairments. Adapted from the stage to the page, *Dementia Man* is a must-read for every medical student. We look forward to many more years of collaboration.

Marc Rothman, MD,
co-founder of Dementia Spring Foundation

Sam Simon offers a deeply personal journey into the escalating effects of cognitive impairment told from the "inside." As someone with Alzheimer's disease, Sam's unique perspective makes for a compelling and engaging story. The power of *Dementia Man: An Existential Journey* lies in Sam's ability to weave his personal story into the broader fabric of society's failure to adequately deal with escalating memory loss and the personality changes wrought by terminal diseases like Alzheimer's.

The book recounts Sam's career as a "professional troublemaker," a role that equips him to chart a courageous course, honestly and publicly describing his experiences both with the disease and the shortcomings of the medical establishment that makes too many assumptions about cognitively impaired patients. *Dementia Man* is rich with anecdotes as Sam bravely tells his story of cognitive decline from "the inside"—from someone actually living the story he tells. He rejects physician-assisted suicide, concentrating instead on life's possibilities even with limitations wrought by a progressive and incurable disease. And his story is told against the backdrop of his lifelong love affair with his wife, Susan, their prior journey with her breast cancer and her role now as a cognitive navigator as Sam continues his existential journey.

Rev. Robert Chase,
founding director of Intersections International

Samuel A. Simon Esq., diagnosed with early-stage Alzheimer's disease, raises his voice against this incurable condition as only a born troublemaker can—by sharing his experiences with the medical establishment, his family and friends, and finally with his own soul as he tries to gain understanding of what's happening to his body and his mind. An advocate for greater knowledge and understanding since his days as a Nader's Raider, Sam describes his frustrations, loneliness, and breakthroughs through this daring memoir. Taking a note from the Book of Deuteronomy, he decides to "choose life" for as long as he has control. This is a book not of heartbreak but of hope that shares one person's journey into what it's like to knowingly enter life's final act.

Francie Schwartz,
senior editor at *Moment* magazine,
author of *Passage to Pesach.*
co-author of *The Jewish Moral Virtues*
and *A Touch of the Sacred*

DEMENTIA MAN

An existential journey

SAMUEL A. SIMON

Dementia Man: An Existential Journey

© Copyright 2025 Samuel A. Simon. All Rights Reserved

All rights reserved. No part of this publication may be reproduced in any form, or by any means, electronic or mechanical, including photocopying, recording, or any information browsing, storage, or retrieval system, without permission in writing from the publisher.

Disclaimer: This is a work of creative non-fiction. All information provided in this book is for general informational and entertainment purposes. The events and conversations in this memoir are true to the best of the author's memory and not a source of medical or other advice. The author and publisher assume no responsibility for errors, inaccuracies, omissions, or any other inconsistencies herein. The medical information and treatments are as recalled by the author, a writer, and should not be viewed as medically accurate either at the time referred to in the book, or as advice or basis for a modern treatment of Alzheimer's. Anyone who suspects they have Alzheimer's or any other illness should seek immediate medical attention by qualified medical personnel.

For more information about this title or to request bulk pricing, visit www.DementiaMan.com.

Paperback ISBN: 978-1-7379097-3-6
eBook ISBN: 978-1-7379097-4-3

Names: Simon, Sam, 1945- author.
Title: Dementia man : an existential journey / Samuel A. Simon.
Description: McLean, Virginia : The Actual Dance, LLC, [2025]
Identifiers: ISBN: 9781737909736 (paperback) | 9781737909743 (ebook)
Subjects: LCSH: Simon, Sam, 1945- | Alzheimer's disease--Patients--Biography. | Medical care--United States. | LCGFT: Autobiographies. | BISAC: HEALTH & FITNESS / Diseases & Conditions / Alzheimer's & Dementia. | BIOGRAPHY & AUTOBIOGRAPHY / Disability. | BIOGRAPHY & AUTOBIOGRAPHY / Memoirs.
Classification: LCC: RC523.2 .S56 2025 | DDC: 362.1968310092--dc23

TABLE OF CONTENTS

Preface..xiii

Introduction xix

CHAPTER 1: In the Beginning: Nothingness 1

CHAPTER 2: Seeking Help and Losing Hope.............. 19

CHAPTER 3: The Gifts of My Parents..................... 35

CHAPTER 4: Existential Training......................... 47

CHAPTER 5: Becoming a Troublemaker 55

CHAPTER 6: Calming Down and Falling in Love 77

CHAPTER 7: A Great Plan Until It Wasn't................. 83

CHAPTER 8: Starting a Career as a Troublemaker 91

CHAPTER 9: Susan's Existential Journey 125

CHAPTER 10: The Alzheimer's Diagnosis Starting
My Existential Journey 135

CHAPTER 11: What To Do Now?........................153

CHAPTER 12: My Changing Reality......................167

Chapter 13: Living My Values as I Die 175

Chapter 14: An Agenda for Change 181

Chapter 15: Last Words 195

Dementia Man Poetry 199

Appendix: Words of Caution 207

Appreciation 217

About the Author..................................... 227

DEDICATION

To those who choose life, even with dementia
To those who care for them
And especially to my LovePartner™
Susan M. Simon
The other half of my whole

PREFACE

You are about to join my journey through a disease that is not yet curable. It is a journey in progress as I write this book. Depending on when you read and finish the book, it may still be underway... or not.

The story is autobiographical. I have chosen to write about myself, not because I am unique. To the contrary, at this time in history, I am one of millions facing cognitive decline or disease as we enter the later stages of our lives. I have been diagnosed with early-stage Alzheimer's. So now, I am simply one guy among two million-plus people with cognitive issues in 2025. We, those of us with some form of cognitive disease, then affect the lives of double or triple that number. Two whole generations of society—baby boomers and their children—are included. It is becoming pervasive, devastating, and impacting millions.

The medical and related support systems are not prepared. Some individuals are driven to suicide as a result, and others, the immediate and extended families of those with the diseases, are driven into poverty, and almost all struggle through a non-transparent, confusing social and medical infrastructure.

My goal in writing and sharing my story is to invite you to join a revolution in reimagining the journey, and implementing urgently needed changes in how people with cognitive disorders are perceived, treated, and supported in our society, as well as how their families and loved ones are supported throughout the process. Perhaps the gift of my diagnosis is that I can help bring about these changes just a bit sooner than might otherwise happen by telling this story on stage and in print.

Of course, I am not the only one with these views or the only one to speak out. Nor am I a doctor, nor am I a psychologist, nor am I an "expert." I am just a guy—someone who has grown up and had a professional career as what I call a "troublemaker." A lawyer and high-profile consumer advocate who transformed into an actor and playwright in later life. I believe that one of the most effective ways to achieve change is through the power of art and theater to influence decision-makers. I am now someone with Alzheimer's Disease. My response to my illness has been to write and perform a one-man play, *Dementia Man: An Existential Journey*, and now this memoir with the same title. My work is often referred to as a "rare patient voice" in a field where most individuals with the disease lose their capacity to engage with the everyday tasks of daily living, much less write a play and get on stage.

It is fair to say that in 2025, people with cognitive decline are most often seen as people incapable of leading meaningful lives. The process of disease progression and its impact on the family are extraordinarily challenging, and often perceived as unbearably tragic for family and society.

It doesn't have to be this way.

I want the world to adapt to us as it has adapted to other people with disabilities. I urge reform in the so-called dementia world, from medicine to social and institutional infrastructures. I hate that word, dementia. One of my advocacy goals is to be a loud voice in the emerging campaign to eliminate that word in the context of people with neurocognitive disorders. I also want the medical world, particularly the neurology world, to change—to align with the family and personal needs of people diagnosed with neurocognitive disorders (the correct medical reference to brain disorders causing cognitive impairment).

I hear repeatedly the same story: "The doctor said we were only going to get worse, and then they sent us off into the world to find our way." That was our experience, Susan's—my wife—and mine. I argue that no neurologist or medical system should be allowed to practice in the field of diagnosing neurocognitive disorders or neurocognitive mental issues without an infrastructure of some sort for patient and family support within the practice or system. When I was initially diagnosed with cognitive impairment, we walked out of the neurologist's office and were told that the doctor had "left no instructions and the office would be in touch if he wanted to see us again." (They never did.)

The disparity between cognitive issues and other serious diseases is enormous. Medicare & Medicaid Services

(CMS), as of January 1, 2024, pays for patient navigation and navigation-related services for breast cancer patients. Yet, for individuals with cognitive disorders, let's say Alzheimer's disease, like me, they do not. The idea isn't even on the table.

I believe there should be cognitive navigators (CNs) available as disability accommodation and an accompanying infrastructure to help us navigate the world and to help us live and engage in life even with our disease, for many years after diagnosis. We have learned that depending on how early in the disease's progression we get diagnosed, it can be as many as five to 10 years before a patient will get a lot worse.

Most importantly, I want to help change the narrative and the imagination about the disease, and in so doing, help individuals with a diagnosis believe and live a life of love, engagement, and meaning for as long as possible. I do that by being loud and proud as I go through a journey I did not choose, as I stand up to make my journey meaningful to me, my loved ones, and the world at large.

I am not the only voice with this message. Throughout my journey today, and through the gift of my work on stage, I have had the opportunity to meet and get to know numerous experts and influential voices in this field. In the appendix, I reference and link to some of those experts and their work. I extend here, and later, my gratitude to all of them and others in this field who share this energy to build a movement of life and living meaningfully as we change.

Sam's Psalm

I walk in the valley of nothingness.

No light. No sound. No smell.
No taste. No feeling.
Infinity has come for me.

Alone in nothing, I am left to wonder.
Am I dead or not?

Then, a tiny spark of light.
An existential moment in the night.
I transform into a new being.

This is how it is and always will be.
A different table is set before me.

Still, I'm filled with all I need. I lack nothing.

You who see the change do not cry.
Your eyes belie the truth.
I am not afraid, and I am not alone.
Still whole, I dwell anew with the Shepherd.
And will for years to come.

INTRODUCTION

It is mid-2022. Susan, my wife, then of 54 ½ years, and I arrive at the office of our neurologist, a Dr. Banks, to receive the results of a PET/CT with contrast of my brain. The issue is my cognitive decline, recently diagnosed as Mild Cognitive Impairment (MCI). The hospital that performed the scan sent the results to our neurologist. Susan and I are looking forward to the appointment. It had been about two years since the MCI diagnosis. Getting the PET/CT with contrast had been a struggle. Our goal has been to find out what is causing my cognitive decline and come up with a treatment plan that will help return me to something close to normal.

We are feeling more relieved than worried. Our journey to this point has been one of the most frustrating periods of our lives—mine and Susan's. The neurological process, as you will read, was excruciatingly long. We had never been exposed to brain issues.

As soon as we get to the front desk, we sense that something is different from our last visit. The desk staff is not chatty. The two women behind the front desk glass look at each other. One picks up a phone to let the doctor know we have arrived. The other person walks around and says, "Come with me." We pass the treatment room doors, three of them, on our left, and we arrive at the door at the end of the hall. She knocks, and without waiting for an answer, opens the door, peeks at the doctor, and motions us in. We settle in our seats.

The neurologist sitting across from us is clearly uncomfortable. He doesn't make eye contact. We are in his private office, not the familiar exam room. I wonder now if we should have realized this was a dramatic moment for both parties—the patient and the doctor.

Dr. Banks is looking down at a piece of paper he has pulled halfway out from inside a brown folder on his lap. "It looks like we are at a new diagnosis," he says in a quiet voice.

He doesn't look up. There is a pause, a hesitation. Then he mumbles: "Early-stage Alzheimer's."

There follows an infinite moment when the universe stops. Silence. My life does not flash in front of me. I don't start to cry. Susan doesn't grab my hand or hug me. We sit in a silence that still comes around occasionally. Indeed, it is as if time itself has stopped.

Today, as I write this book, about seven years into this journey, I think back on that moment and wonder if that silence was because we didn't know much about Alzheimer's. Or because we did. I only remember the silence.

I was fortunate to be "early stage" when first diagnosed. Indeed, Dr. Banks told us at that appointment it could take 10 to 15 years before things got "a lot worse." I was 76 at the time. In retrospect, I could have dismissed it, thinking something else would get me by then. "So what?" As I have thought about it, I realize that there were symptoms for years before even seeing a doctor, and, as you will read, it had been three years earlier that I had been diagnosed with Mild Cognitive Impairment. So, at that point, I wonder, "Years from when?" It is now, as I write, ten or more years since I noticed all this starting, and I can tell that my symptoms are progressing.

In the days, weeks, and early months following the diagnosis of early-stage Alzheimer's, I struggled to come to terms with the existential questions that surround a terminal diagnosis. "What should I do? What are my options?" Those questions are still on my mind.

My heart and soul were all twisted up as I initially dealt with these questions. "Can I continue in this new life of mine—or do I need to curl up and die?" When I told my internist of my diagnosis, he gave me a book on Alzheimer's and suggested I see HIS psychiatrist (who didn't take insurance and charged $400 an hour). The *New York Times* recently published an exposé on the author of that book, labeling him a quack.

Even now, my family and friends are empathetic, yet I still see the terror in their eyes and sense it in their hearts as they react to the news. I hear the subtext of their reactions, "Oh my God! That is terrible. What a horrible disease. You poor thing." Or more descriptive: "You poor thing! My mother had it and was walking around the house not knowing where she was and who we were. Then we put her in a memory unit."

I wonder if those people understand the impact of their words on me—if they appreciate the discomfort and added weight to the burden of knowing what comes from watching their faces and hearing the terror in their voices. No wonder so many people with the diagnosis fold into themselves and never come out. Or worse, end their lives through some form of suicide.

My impulse to do something different, including writing this book, comes from two places. One is Susan's strength and unconditional love. She had her turn in my skin. She is an unlikely survivor of advanced breast cancer. Her experience, her journey from a presumed end-of-life illness to unlikely survivorship, reminds both of us that even when the doctors say, "It's over," it is still possible to beat the odds or otherwise be a statistical outlier in the medical journey. Having gone through Susan's brush with death is the primary source of my belief that I, too, might be an "outlier"—the 1 percent or maybe the only one—who beats the odds on this disease. Whatever that phrase may mean for Alzheimer's.

Another source of encouragement was and is my professional artistic cohort in what I now refer to as the *Fourth Age* of my life. It began around my 60th year, as I transitioned from being a lawyer, businessperson, and advocate to an actor, playwright, and solo performer. I went from what my son once described as a "minor public celebrity" in the Washington, DC, policy world to a playwright, author, and self-producing artist. My first experience in this new period of my life was to write a play (*The Actual Dance*) and then a book (by the same title) about Susan's breast cancer and her brush with an end-of-life diagnosis.

I had been immersed in this new—fourth age—era of my life for nearly seven years when I received my earliest diagnosis of cognitive decline: Mild-Cognitive Impairment or "MCI" in 2018. As I started letting my professional theatrical colleagues know about my diagnosis, the first words were: "Write about it. Live the story on the page and on the stage." This advice wasn't obvious to me, and I was incredulous. Yet they persisted, even when they learned that my decline was attributable to Alzheimer's disease. You will read names in the acknowledgment of many of those positive voices. This work, and the play by the same name, is the result.

As you'll read in the pages that follow, I have come to learn and believe that life with this disease is worth living, every single day of it, up until its natural conclusion. Indeed, now, as I enter my eighth decade of life and face other medical issues, prostate cancer, for example, I realize my end may indeed be caused by something different.

The play and this book are also a story of becoming—becoming different, defying norms, and aspiring to an experience that defies stereotypes and expectations.

The feedback we—Susan and I—get most often at the end of a performance of the play is that I am "brave." The word perplexes me. My brother-in-law, a retired Major General (Army), recently completed his autobiography and shared an insight about what constitutes "bravery." His context was battlefield combat, and he observed that bravery comes if, and only if, you are first afraid and still move into danger. He argues that just moving into danger unafraid isn't brave. Well, I am not and have not been afraid. Oddly, my initial reaction was curiosity. A poem I wrote not long after being diagnosed, which you can read on page 201, concluded with the question: "I wonder what the Sam of me then will know of the Sam of me now."

So, I'm not brave by this definition, since I am not afraid, and I don't feel brave now or ever have in this process. Truthfully, I don't always know what I feel. I am uncertain sometimes. I am angry sometimes, not because I have the disease. I am outraged at how the medical and social infrastructure of this country is failing people like me. Most often, my feelings are familiar, consistent with how I have confronted every step of my life's journey, the person who always speaks out and challenges norms and practices that he perceives as unfair or unjust. I use the label "troublemaker" to express that life history. Causing trouble for me is speaking out for a world of meaning, justice, and love for all people. In some ways, I experience my own life story as doing just that, defying my own expectations along the way.

In reading this story, I hope you, too, might come to defy your expectations and imagine the future differently. For everyone. As I write in the play and talk about here, I have seen the world change in ways no one could have imagined. Earlier in my lifetime—and perhaps yours—there were no people in wheelchairs on our streets, theaters did not have captioning, and we could not fathom a blind person sitting in the audience of a play. Yet this is now the norm, though there is still much more to be done in even the near future.

One last note about "the end." There is another movement afoot, sometimes called euthanasia or assisted or accompanied suicide. The movement promotes the laws that create legal systems for people to choose when and how to die. Advocates for this cause often claim that aided or assisted suicide, which, as of this writing, is legal in eleven states and Washington, DC, provides greater agency and is more humane than the journey through a long, expensive, and sometimes painful illness. My call here, to those of us going through cognitive changes and to our loved ones, is to reimagine the future.

Aspire to a future where it is possible for all of us, however we present ourselves, to live meaningful lives. A world in which the people and systems adapt, and we all commit to taking life's journey to its natural end, together, if not for ourselves, then for those generations yet to come.

CHAPTER 1

IN THE BEGINNING: NOTHINGNESS

There is a place that exists for me that I could not have imagined and which I have never understood. Not a dream, though it is like sleep. In the moment, it is not a hallucination, though that becomes debatable.

It is a mental state of timeless nothingness. I eventually name it: "The Nothingness Place." I speak of it as though it is a physical place because for a period of time in my disease journey, I would, while in full awareness, slip from "normal" into what I would experience as nothingness.

I speak of this in the present tense, though as you will read, medication has halted this phenomenon, at least for the moment. Yet, I often feel I am on the precipice. When I exit into the nothingness, it is a moment in time when I mentally leave the "real world." I have no idea how long I am "gone." I intuit that perhaps it typically lasts a nanosecond or two, or even less, since no one around me seems to notice. For me, though, it feels like forever. I wonder if there are two modalities of existence. A physical, real-world time in which I am physically and cognitively present. Then there are times when I am physically present, that is, visibly present to others, though cognitively, I am somewhere or perhaps even something else.

I experience infinity as a place or a moment in which there is no light, even though I have eyes. No sound, even though I have ears. No smell, no taste, no feeling, no touch. Still, at that moment, I will sense my feet move, though not even touch a floor. It is as if I float in infinity. Outer space comes to mind. Maybe even tumbling through dark nothingness.

Is it "real?" Was it real? As I just wrote, this is where it becomes debatable. I was once asked that question by a medical student—a neurology intern—who was present in an exam room observing my cognitive evaluation by a neurologist. The intern heard me try to describe "The Nothingness Place."

"Is it real or a hallucination?" she asked.

My immediate response: "It's real!" Then I realized the only thing that was "real" at that moment was my sense of being cognitively in this state of obliviousness, that there was no other actual place, or another place measurable or present for anyone else. It was a cognitive event for me. As real as this nothingness is and has been to me in my "momentary reality," in the objective world, it is a hallucination. Though at times, I want to argue that if it is what I am experiencing, it is, by definition, "real."

When I go to that place or state, when I exit the "normal world" into that infinity, I am aware that I am there. I scream internally for a door, or an "other side," for reality. Sometimes. I think this is what death might be like. Yet I can sense I am not dead, and of course, somehow, I come out and confirm that I am not—yet—dead.

Whatever that place might be these days, it is just me with symptoms of a cognitive impairment, eventually to be diagnosed as Alzheimer's Disease.

The Road to Nothingness

It started as momentary memory lapses. The forgetfulness bothered me, though it was not at all like what eventually developed. It was more of an irritation, and it didn't occur to me to see a doctor. The first time I said anything to a doctor was toward the end of a routine annual physical with my then-longtime internist. Now, almost 30 years later, I can picture the moment in my head as clearly as if it were yesterday. He has finished the EKG, I am rebuttoning my shirt, and at that moment, it pops into my head to complain about my memory. I believe I was in my mid-to-late 50s at the time.

He almost guffaws. "Sam, I've known you a long time, and there is nothing wrong with **your** memory!" Then, almost as a throw away note to emphasize his point, "Now, if you can't remember what you ate for breakfast, then maybe there could be a problem."

He moves along, writing notes, checking files, ignoring me as I close my eyes and try to picture the morning breakfast table. I have no frigging idea what I had for breakfast just a few hours ago. I do picture the kitchen in my mind, unsure what chair I'd sat in or anything in front of me. I get his attention and stutter, "Uh, I have no idea what I had for breakfast this morning." He refers me to a psychologist, not a neurologist. In retrospect, he must have thought I was depressed.

Indeed, he had known me for nearly 25 years. When we started, I worked for Ralph Nader and was often on television. I authored a book and gave him a signed copy. I might have been his highest-profile Washington, DC, patient.

At the time I complained to him about my memory, I was president of a highly successful consulting firm called Issue Dynamics, Inc., or IDI for short. Our mission was to build bridges between consumer advocates and corporations for win-win solutions, and, at the time, I had received a lot of publicity around our innovative approaches.

In fact, by the time of this appointment, the doctor could have seen me on local or national news programs such as Face the Nation, the Today Show, all the evening news shows, and even the Phil Donahue or Oprah Winfrey shows. I suspect these media appearances were factors in his conclusion that I must be under a lot of stress.

I make an appointment with the psychologist he recommends. The psychologist administers a brief memory test and discusses my job and career with me for a bit. He then prescribes an antidepressant, Wellbutrin. I am not sure I'm depressed, though I'm under a lot of pressure and doing a lot of work at my growing firm. I am also getting restless, wanting to do something more in life. Then I find out, again, that I am not so different from other colleagues who run small businesses. I have been a member of an organization called TEC—a national company that sets up local roundtables—regular meetings—of CEOs of small businesses, like mine, to network with each other. It allows me to talk to other people, mostly men, who, like me, work alone at the top of a growing small business. At the next meeting of my group, following that session with the psychologist, I learn that three other CEOs in our group take Wellbutrin. "It's not depression," I think, "it's just the anxiety of running a company. I am normal!"

The feeling, though, of trying to recall what I had for breakfast—the void and infinite nothingness of my mind as I try to remember what I had for breakfast in that moment—sticks with me. It lingers in the background of what slowly and over time becomes a pattern of forgetting and confusion. Mostly moments and little things. Often directions. "Just normal aging memory loss, I guess." This is what family and friends suggest when I mention something about forgetting things.

I don't know if the gap between this first "worrying" in my late 50s is related to where I am now in my late 70s. That moment 25 plus years ago in my internist's office isn't the only time I worried about my memory as I got older. Memory concerns as people age seem routine, even normal. The question is how can we know when they are not just normal aging, or if they might be symptoms of something much worse—like Alzheimer's disease?

Another earlier "moment" that stands out as I look back is what happened on the trip Susan and I took to attend Susan's niece's wedding in Austin, Texas. We had lived in

Austin for three years when I was in law school, albeit 30 years or so earlier. The town had changed more than I imagined. Driving from the hotel to the event venue requires Susan's help directing me with the AAA map. The next day, though, it is worse. It's as if I had never driven the route, even though I had done so the previous evening to the same destination. For me, everything has changed. It's the same map, yet seemingly a different Sam. It is frustrating for Susan, and I keep telling her, "I don't care what the map says; I have never been on this route before!" I am shouting at her to look closer at the map and ensure we aren't lost. Of course, we aren't.

It bothers both of us, yet we let it go. We have a 'spat' and move on. We get to the party and have a good time.

My suddenly suspect directional skills do not improve. After years of traveling—and finding my way—to places I've never been to, I now get lost in my own neighborhood. Not only do I get lost, but I also get confused about navigating what had been familiar intersections. For example, a traffic circle is a few miles from our home. It isn't on a typical route, and I don't remember why, at that moment, I needed to go there, nor why I needed to get some gasoline in the car. We have a different regular gas station. Whatever the reason, the Texaco station is on the edge of the traffic circle and easy enough to "enter." After getting five gallons to last until the regular gas fill-up, I try to drive out back onto the traffic circle. Except, I find myself driving in circles around the Texaco gas station property, desperately trying to figure out how to get myself onto the road on the right side of a traffic circle. I lose count of how many times I go around, maybe five or maybe six times. Around and around. I cannot figure it out. I finally noticed a different exit at the rear of the gas station that leads into a connected shopping mall parking lot. I take this back exit from the Texaco station into the shopping mall lot; from there, a rear-mall exit onto a regular two-lane road that leads up to a traffic light at the circle. I now enter the traffic circle at the traffic light. Again, I don't obsess about the frustrating moment, though the incident bothers me. I let it go, sort of.

About this time, there are some changes in our, Susan's, and my medical world. We had never seen the same internist. My long-term internist—the fellow who referred me to a psychologist when I first complained about memory, had become ill with cancer, and stopped seeing patients for a while. Susan's primary internist started reducing the size of her practice. So, we decided to see the same new internal medicine doctor. While he is a younger man, he specializes in older patients, "geriatrics," though we don't see ourselves as *that* old. Well, I guess we were because it was around 2015, and we were both 70.

At some point in the process of the new doctor getting to know me, I tell him about my memory concerns and that I had taken Wellbutrin. I explained that I continue getting frustrated and occasionally confused around names, places, and directions. He administers what is called a "mini-mental" exam. A few questions, remembering a list of words. I guess I do okay on the tests because he reacts by telling me that nothing that I described sounds different to him than what happens as part of normal aging. Everyone's memory gets worse as they age, he explains. And the quick test he administered didn't send up any red flags. What do I know? I had never been "old" before.

As 2015 comes to an end, I begin to experience more changes that, in retrospect, I believe were signs of an already present cognitive issue. It is hard for me now, as I write this book about this disease, to remember the exact sequence of events. What is here is generally accurate, and what I do remember—the brightest moments—are clear, just not exactly when they happened in relation to other things that happened in my life, if you know what I mean.

The Nothingness Place became very specific. I don't remember the very first time it happened. I remember my slow realization that what was happening was not normal and indeed alarming. Typically, I'm sitting down trying to remember a specific fact—date, place, name, event, schedule, whatever. I close my "real eyes," and then the real "I," Sam, vanishes. Then, a miniature pair of eyes—maybe just eyeballs—take over the hunt for the "fact." These mini eyes sit just inside (behind) my forehead, internal to and above my actual eyes. I am able to see or sense these tiny eyes. It is like seeing myself from inside myself.

These two miniature eyes inside my brain look to the right of where I face. Always to the right, for some reason. (I am right-handed; I wonder if that's part of it.) It is as if my brain somehow controls the eyes of my mind to look for the piece of information that exists in the abyss that has formed off to the right. You have to understand that at that moment, the answers to *everything* are somewhere off to the right in my brain or head. I just need to penetrate the void, the blackness, the infinity between me and the answer. My pain is in the search, wanting to know so badly whatever it is I am searching for and not being able to find it—not knowing in that instant whether I am dead or alive.

Yet the only vision these fictitious eyes of my mind can "see" or experience is an infinite void. In my world, in those moments, "nothing" is black because there is nothingness. I think of it as a "color," though I am eventually reminded that "black" is *not* a color. As I write this, it feels like a circular truism, just as I felt it at the time. Around and around and around. Black infinite nothingness and the awareness that I urgently need to find something, but it is nothing and around again.

The experience is of me floating, moving, or tumbling in infinite deep space. Yet, all the while, I'm sitting somewhere in the real world, about to respond to a question, or write a word, type on a keyboard, or make an argument. In my "reality," I can't act. I am frozen in this deep-space-like plane of existence, trying to connect the synapses that enable me to respond to the requirement. I remember wondering during the transitional—liminal—moment of traveling back to the "real world," if I am, in fact, dead and that "death" itself might be liminal.

Sadly, I never find the answers I am looking for in those moments. When I return to the present, I know where I have been—nowhere, the infamous Nothingness Place. I am bothered and worried, and do not know what to do or how to react. I just hope it won't happen again. You see, I can forget and not know things in this reality. I don't have to always go into Nothingness to forget. It is seemingly a random disappearance.

It is now 2016, and more alarming incidents have emerged. I can't remember every one of them anymore, forgive me. I mainly recall only the brightest, frightening events. For example, the first time I remember driving on the wrong side of the road was one day back when I am still working. I leave my office in downtown Washington, DC, for a business meeting that is on the fourth floor of an office building in Arlington, Virginia. When the meeting ends, I casually walk to the elevator and press the #1 button with the star beside it. I rely heavily on the "star" now to prevent me from going to random lower floors that use the "1" as opposed to B, (basement) or M (Mezzanine), which is considered in some buildings to be the main floor. Once the door opens, I step out of the elevator, walk down the hallway to the main door, exit, and walk into the parking lot to get in my car—all perfectly routine.

Yes, it takes me a few minutes to find my car, though at that time, that seems typical. Today, in 2025, I am deep into the phase of getting old. No matter where I am, whenever I leave a store or a building to a parking area, I freeze. I close my eyes and try to picture where I parked my car, and then I give up trying to remember and resort to walking up and down the lanes in the lot. Yes, I know I can hit the button on my key fob and make the car honk; it just never seems to work when I need it to.

Okay. There have even been a time or two when I've needed to locate a garage parking attendant and plead for help. It is so embarrassing and a bit frightening. Did you know the parking attendants in some places have little golf carts available to drive us forgetful people around to locate our cars when the worst happens? I now take pictures of the parking space and any signs indicating the floor and space. Sometimes, pictures help.

Anyway, finding my car on this particular day is not too difficult. I get in, pull out of the space, drive up to the parking lot exit lane, turn right, and drive up to a stop sign at the entry to the main road. I stop and look both ways. I don't see any cars coming, so I pull out and turn to the left. Suddenly, there are car honks from every direction. At first, I don't realize the honking is about me. As I drive up the road, I look up ahead and notice that at the traffic light at the next intersection, four cars are turning into my traffic lane. Boom! I'm awake! Yikes, I am on the wrong side of the road. I do an urgent U-turn. It scares the crap out of me, and I wonder, "How the hell did that happen?"

Yet, when I tell friends and family about the incident, typically all I get is, "Oh, I've done that too." At first, those "me too" reassurances calm me down. These "small" lapses seem like inconsequential "oopses." I probably am just not paying close attention in my "old age." At that time, I'm commuting every other week to work in New York City as a Senior Fellow at a non-profit. It means I'm pretty "with it" most of the time. Heck, if I can figure out how to commute and live in New York every other week, I must be damned normal. Indeed, today, every time I tell this story on stage, just like when it happened back then, I get the same reaction: dozens of audience members shake their heads, signaling that they, too, have had the same experience—driving on the wrong side of the road.

The next memorable event for me is something different. It is several months later, a Friday at noon. At the time, I had been having lunch every Friday for about five years at the same local restaurant in McLean, Virginia, with my friend and rabbi, Rabbi Laszlo Berkowits, also known as Larry. We lost him in 2021.

I could write an entire book about Larry and me. Maybe I should, if I still have the cognitive capacity. It's one of those things about being "in-between," with a cognitive disease, we are still able to regret things yet undone. He wrote his autobiography, though, with my help. You should get his book: *The Boy Who Lost His Birthday* (Hamilton Books, 2008).

Our Larry was about 17 years older than me, so we could have been brothers. Heck, Susan is 17 years younger than her oldest sister, and my oldest sister was nine years older than me.

We met in 1973, when our family—Susan, me, and our two infant kids—joined the Reform Jewish temple in Falls Church, Virginia, where he was rabbi, Temple Rodef Shalom. Typical of me in those days, I didn't just become another member; I became active in all sorts of programs and occasionally sounded off about how things needed to be changed, and boy, did I get noticed. At the time, even though I was a new member, I spoke out at a congregational meeting to complain about how they weren't asking people to pay enough toward a new building campaign. Talk about Chutzpah! I hadn't even pledged yet; I was so new!

Over the years, we became active in the temple, and in 1980, when I was 35 years old, I was elected president of the congregation. Susan became president in 1996. It meant we spent a lot of time at the temple and with the rabbi and his family—his wife Judy and their two children.

Larry and I became unlikely best friends over the 48 years we knew each other. We became remarkably close in the '80s and '90s, and stayed that way until 2021, the year he passed away. In the early 2000s, in the period right after his wife, Judy, passed away, I became the rabbi's travel companion back to Germany, where at 16 years old, he was a prisoner in the Auschwitz (in Poland) death camp. Back then, while in Auschwitz, he tricked the Germans into believing he was able (at 16 years old) to work on trucks, so they sent him and his friends to a truck factory in Germany. From there, as it became apparent Germany was losing the war, he was transported with other kids to a POW camp called Wöbbelin, adjacent to a small town, Ludwigslust; it was at Wöbbelin where, as a 17-year-old boy, he was liberated by the 82nd Airborne. Larry and I traveled together to all those places several times over the next few years.

After Larry's retirement as senior rabbi in 1998, he and I developed this Friday lunch ritual—okay lunch routine—at the McLean Family Restaurant (MFR for short), which is only a quarter mile from our respective homes. "If it's Friday, Sam and Larry are at McLean Family," became a thing among our various family and friend circles. Sometimes, folks would show up and join us or just say hello.

On this particular Friday, after lunch, I get into my car to take the short drive home, and I suddenly lose cognitive awareness. Mentally, it is as if I am floating down the street in a machine as it glides down the road. I am a spectator, not a driver. The street signs and building signs float out in front of me, seeming to dance in the sky. The white letters of words on the small green street signs with the name of a street I've never heard of make no sense to me.

I can close my eyes today, as I write this, and recall— almost feel— looking up and around at street signs as the machine (aka car) moves forward and wondering, *Where is that? Where am I?* When I put my head down and look ahead, I hallucinate, believing that the 7-11 store sign is now sitting on the hood of my car, facing my windshield. I am confused, panicked, and sense that something is terribly wrong.

As I reflect on that moment, I don't understand how I could be totally "out of it" yet seemingly in control of the car. Thank goodness no one was hurt. Yet, even now, sitting here writing, I close my eyes and return to that moment, sitting in that floating machine, recalling the surprise as I somehow recognize a turn lane ahead, confused. Perhaps it is the familiarity of the corner Exxon Station and its bright red and white colors that brings me back to some sense of reality. Enough to recognize the turn lane. Or maybe it is the outsized traffic signal—outsized to me in my brain—with a bright green turn arrow. It is as if the traffic signal is trying to catch my attention. It is abnormally high, seemingly unconnected to the rest of the streetlight structure (the yellow and red), and is very large. There is bright yellow metal around the big dark glass, inside of which a giant green arrow is yelling at me, "Turn-left stupid!"

I do what the voice in my head tells me to do. I move forward into the intersection and turn left onto the far side of the cross street. I pull up to the opposite curb and stop. I put the car into park. I close my eyes and take deep breaths. When I open them, the world has returned to normal. I drive home very, very slowly. I don't tell anyone about what has just happened.

Despite all these events, I don't sense there is anything seriously wrong with me. I can be frustrated when they happen, and yet, based on all the "I do that too" responses I get, I continue to buy into the "normal aging" mantra that I have been getting from my internist. Every time I complain about memory—I don't call it cognition, I don't even know that word yet—my internist keeps telling me not to worry, it's just "normal aging."

Perhaps I'm just in denial and too busy to let them bother me too much. On the other hand, perhaps I sense something is seriously wrong, and that is why I don't tell anyone about this most recent incident.

The Turning Point

The turning point in the journey, the tipping point that triggers me to seek help, is something new and weird. It is an escalation of the Nothingness experience, though I haven't started using that term yet. At this point, I still don't have a name for this moment of confusion. Compared to the driving moments, slipping into blankness seems almost irrelevant. The "blankness event," if you will, seems always to take place in the moment of trying to remember a name, date, or place. Typically, I would be sitting at a desk or on the computer, or in a room with someone, having a conversation. It bothers me, yet it does not scare me. Mostly it frustrates me, perhaps an omen of what will develop later—something known as Alzheimer's agitation.

The experiences begin to intensify over the next few months. The most vivid escalation event is the day I head to the local pharmacy inside the Giant grocery store to fill a prescription. The Giant, our local grocery store, is only a short one-minute drive from our house. I park the car, walk into the store, and down an aisle to the pharmacy. I am second in line. Then I disappear.

I do not remember walking up to the counter. It is as if a button is pushed, next, and in an instant, my consciousness is whooshed into an infinite opaque expanse. It is indeed as if I am floating in deep space. So far away that there is no light, no sound, no feeling—there is just Nothingness. Absolutely Nothing! I'm not sleeping because I'm aware of Nothing. I am not hearing because there is no sound in Nothing. Yet I am aware I am in Nothing. Does this sound confusing to you? Damned right.

In that infinite moment in the drugstore, though, apparently standing mute and silent, I suddenly hear something that sounds like a voice. "How may I help you, sir?" At first, the remote echoing of the voice in my head makes me wonder if the sound is real. I have no sense of a corporeal self—of reality—and I don't know where I am or what I am, until a second sound. This time, more clearly, a voice from in front of me repeats the question with more energy and quite a few more decibels. Almost a shout, "HOW MAY I HELP YOU, SIR?"

Suddenly, I realize that this is real. Still confused, I stutter: "Uh."

The pharmacist standing in front of me, behind a small counter, now seems to realize something might be wrong. She changes her demeanor entirely. She leans toward me, speaks softly, and repeats, "Excuse me, sir, are you dropping off or picking up a prescription?" It's like coming out of a hangover. I shake my foggy head, look down at my hand, and notice a prescription. I stick out my hand with the piece of paper for the pharmacist, "Oh, dropping off, sorry."

The experience repeats itself. It can happen at any time and anywhere, and there seems to be no specific cause or trigger. It feels random. Even on a Saturday evening at home, Susan and I are supposed to go to dinner with our friends, Sylvia and Irv, whom we've known for 25 years. Dinner this Saturday at their apartment is part of a monthly routine of getting together, alternating between their place and ours.

So, this Saturday, Susan and I are sitting in the living room, doing whatever; I don't remember anything because I'm only physically sitting in the living room. In that specific moment, just like the moment at the drugstore in line at the pharmacy, my mental self is floating out in the middle of deep space. I can barely make out Susan's words—it's as if they take light years to reach me. It sounds something like: "Time to get ready, Sam."

I have no idea what she means. Ready for what? I'm getting pretty good at reacting in ways that hide my confusion. I stutter, "Whe … wheh … where are we going, Susan? Do I need a tie?"

She stops whatever she is doing, looks over at me, and makes a face—perhaps a sneer? "Sam, it is dinner with Sylvia and Irv at their apartment. We talked about it an hour ago. Get your butt in gear. Get a move on it!"

Transporting from a normal, routine moment in life into this full eclipse of time, light, and space scares and confuses me. At this point in my cognitive journey, I always return to reality when the moment passes. Eventually, a new medication—an antidepressant—is prescribed by my internist to help with my disappearances in Nothingness. The medicine does work to diminish these disappearances. Even then, I continue to live between my own cognitive eclipses.

CHAPTER 2

SEEKING HELP AND LOSING HOPE

These moments of getting lost and falling into infinity eventually become part of our lives, really my life—flipping in and out of The Nothingness Place, as I call it, over and over and over again. Everything is normal, and then, boom, my mind and my body seem to separate. I am simultaneously in two places at the same time, or even in between. Time, mind, and physical space intertwine!

Materially, I can be in front of a pharmacist or in a room with Susan, or even on the subway. I sometimes forget where and when to get off. It is usually the screeching of the train's metal that "wakes me up," so to speak. I'll get off, shake it off, realize where I am, and then get on the next train to my intended stop—or switch to the opposite side of the tracks to get a train in the opposite direction, back a stop or two, to my intended destination. In those moments, I exit the present and am transported to The Nothingness Place.

What finally triggers me to action is my concern, my anxiety, and my sense that something might be terribly wrong with me. Oddly, given Susan and I have been married about 56 years at this point, I am unable—or unwilling—to articulate the nature of the concern. I do not have the words, yet, and I harbor a suspicion she won't understand. I am scared. I can't sleep, I can't talk about it, even with Susan. I know I need help. I finally decide to make an appointment to see my internist.

At first, he too seems frustrated. I detect a "Here he goes again" attitude as I try to explain how things are different from the last time I complained about my memory. Then, I tell him about The Nothingness Place experience, and he immediately perks up. He starts probing, asking me to clarify when and what happens.

He then schedules an appointment for me with his favorite neurology practice.

This reaction triggers an even greater sense that something might be very, very wrong with me. My only experience with a neurologist had been four decades earlier, when I went through treatment for cluster vascular migraine headaches (often described as creating the most severe pain known to humans). I sometimes wonder now if those headaches had anything to do with my Alzheimer's. The neurologists were helpful and pleasant. Except that it was 41 years earlier, and I wasn't thinking about the headaches now, I was just desperate to find out what was going on with me.

With this referral, a brand-new pattern begins to develop—waiting time. Although my internist is the one who called and requested the appointment, the first available time is not for several months. It turns out that the neurologist my internist recommended wasn't available before that. A different one was available earlier, a Doctor Howard. I grabbed that appointment. "Only" two months from now. The wait feels like forever.

I don't remember why I was going to these appointments alone. I do not think Susan or anyone else believes my "slips" or mistakes are anything serious. I suspect they also think I am just overreacting, though they never admit it.

We all look for an explanation. Several years earlier, Susan had watched me go through sleep challenges. At the time, we all attributed them to anxiety around my work. I had been taking sleeping pills every night, and both my earlier doctor and the new one believed that sleep is very important. For a long time, back then, I rarely slept for more than four hours a night. Even on the sleeping pills, a typical night was about five or five and a half hours. Maybe that was why my "memory" was so bad. We were not yet familiar with the phrase *cognitive impairment*. Still, now, I know something is not right.

Even today, as I write this book, it is almost impossible to explain to others how the memory "incidents" and "lapses" have changed. Changed from just "normal aging" to symptoms of something much more serious.

How to accommodate those changes?

Yes, we have established the "designated place" for keys, wallets, and a few other things, yet that doesn't always work. When the keys aren't where they are supposed to be, it's anyone's guess where they might be, and the long hunt is on—as well as the frustration and short tempers. Recently, someone suggested, and I agree, that the difference is that today I can't be prompted, nor can I retrace my steps to remember. The difference between "not finding keys" for an "unimpaired person"—like Susan—and for me is that she can retrace her steps and find the keys. Me, I start searching everywhere. I don't have a place to start because I don't remember where I have been, where the last place "is."

Everything I do seems to take more and more time. It frustrates me to no end. My current internist prescribed a new drug that he just read about, and that in Europe is "off-label" for help with cognitive impairment, which is also an antidepressant. I hesitate, reminded of the earlier incident when my former internist thought I was depressed after I couldn't remember what I had eaten for breakfast that morning and then referred me to the psychologist. This new pill does not improve my memory. I still can't remember the things I can't recall—the ones I was looking for when those two miniature eyes in my brain turned right and carried me into outer space. Still, I am glad I don't resist because since taking it, I have not disappeared into The Nothingness Place.

Occasionally, I can get a sense of being on the precipice of darkness and brace myself. I haven't fallen into it again, thankfully. I wonder, though, when and if I fall, disappear, into The Nothingness Place—infinity—again, I might not come out. I still can imagine a future me sitting in a room in a memory unit of an assisted living center, staring blankly into space.

Pardon all these digressions. It's what you do when you wait and wait for these pending appointments. Finally, the eight weeks are up, and I arrive for my first appointment with Dr. Howard, the neurologist. First visits to any doctor, I suspect, are a bit different. A new building, finding a place to park for the first time, figuring out the elevator, where to turn on the floor when I get to the right floor, a different waiting room, and, of course, waiting. I look around and try to judge whether it is a good place, a bad place, or something in between.

I am invited into a small treatment room, and I wait for about fifteen more minutes. Dr. Howard seems almost bored while I talk about forgetting things and the driving issues. Then I tell him about The Nothingness Place. As I share the sense of looking to the right inside my brain and falling into deep space with awareness, yet no air, sound, or light, I feel that I am traveling through infinite nothingness. I see myself and experience myself at the same time. It is confusing!

Dr. Howard reacts by taking out a pencil and a prescription pad. He immediately begins to schedule me for every electronic study of the brain that exists: a sleep study, an MRI of the brain, and EEG (electroencephalogram) studies up the gazoo. Then, he prescribes a neuropsychological exam, the gold standard for cognitive testing. I never heard the phrase "neuropsychology." It turns out that this particular exam is five hours long. It takes six long months to get through all these exams, most of which I do on my own. I have never had a sleep study before, and I am still unsure what my sleep has to do with my memory. Heck, they even let me take my sleeping pill for the night of the sleep study, which is in a small room inside the medical offices. I wear an oxygen mask, too. I wake up in the morning, get dressed, and drive home—routine. Or so it seems.

The process is roughly the same for all the other studies. It is all strange and new, but not alarming. In retrospect, it is not hard to understand why Susan never joined me for any of these appointments. There was no real alarm in our lives over what was happening; Susan was still working, and so was I. The rest of our lives seemed normal(ish).

The most challenging test is that five-hour neuropsychological exam.

The neuropsychologist's practice, it turns out, is in a building adjacent to Dr. Howard's offices. It's an easy trip, though I recall feeling a bit lonely as I enter his office. The test is administered by three different staff members, not the neuropsychologist. Each person administers a different part of the test. I am quite anxious throughout the test because it is all new. The start of each succeeding part of the test set off my anxiety again. *Now what?* I think and wonder how I will do on this latest section.

I still remember the hardest parts. A list of words is read to me several times, and then later in the exam, I have to recall them. Then there is the part of the test when I have to count backward from 100 by 7s until I am told to stop. ($100 - 7 = 93$ etc.). Boy, do I flop. Next, I have to draw. I am asked to copy various shapes I am shown. I have always had poor handwriting and could never draw well. Not sure how they grade these things. Then, I'm told a story, and an hour later, I am asked to repeat it. I don't recall the story during this first test. Later, after years of taking the exact same test dozens of times, I do better, though I still do terribly on the word-recall portion. In the end, I walk out worried.

It takes eight weeks for the results to be ready. I was expecting to hear from the neurologist. Instead, the neuropsychologist calls to tell me that the results are in, and he can send them to Dr. Howard, or if I am interested, he has an opening and would be happy to provide them to me. All of the tests I went through are on my mind, and I am desperate to get at least some results. I haven't heard from Dr. Howard, and this doctor has an opening in three days! "Yes," I almost scream.

I arrive for the appointment, and we meet in his office, not an exam room. He hands me a 15-page report full of medical jargon, then guides me to the last page and directs my attention to the conclusion: I have MCI. I am Mildly Cognitively Impaired. "What does that mean?" I ask. I've never heard of the phrase, well, not in this context. Ironically, in my other professional life, I am widely known as the man who helped MCI Communications Corporation—known familiarly simply as MCI—the first alternative long-distance company to compete against AT&T in America. I then helped break up the AT&T monopoly. I was the lawyer for all the consumer groups who argued for breaking up AT&T, a position supported by MCI. My brief on the consumer groups was widely quoted in the judge's decision and the press. At about the same time, I wrote a book called *Reverse the Charges, How to Save Money on Your Phone Bill* (Pantheon, 1983), which MCI, the corporation, loved. Ironic, isn't it? I still remember a few lunches I had with Bill McGowen, the then-president of MCI ... the corporation. Those are the days, as I said, when my son saw me as a "minor celebrity." Okay, again, I digress.

The neuropsychologist explains to me that the test I took is standard and based on very specific factors, including my age, gender, education level, nationality, and other elements I don't recall. I am compared to everyone else who is "just like me," that is, those who share these exact same traits. So, my "score," or however the results are interpreted, classifies me, compared to a norm tied to me, as "mildly cognitively impaired." I have MCI. The neuropsychologist doesn't seem upset or worried, and he doesn't suggest any reason or cause for my MCI. He just wishes me well.

I leave his office with a copy of the test results in my hand, still unsure of what it means. Yet, I am delighted! I walk out of the door to their practice, into a hallway, and pump my fist, thinking, "Yes, there is something wrong with me. I am NOT normal. I am not making this stuff up!"

I share the report with Susan when I get home, and she joins the worrying team. She does not seem or act alarmed, even if she is, and I now think I should have someone with me at the doctors' appointments. We both understand that something is wrong. I am not just getting old. She is apologetic about not being able to be with me for these early appointments and gladly joins me at future ones.

We now wait for a few more weeks for the results from all the other tests to come in—the sleep study and all the EEG studies.

Finally, a call from Dr. Howard's office informs us that the results are in and an appointment is available to review them. We look forward to finding out precisely what it all means. What is causing my MCI? Are there any other issues? Most of all, we eagerly anticipate receiving a firm diagnosis, a treatment plan, and a path for me to return to normal.

It has taken months to get to this point, and now it will take another six weeks for the appointment. Yes, six more weeks! It is becoming the rhythm of my and our lives. Six more weeks, six more weeks.

When we arrive, Susan and I are taken into an examination room. It is a 20-minute wait before Dr. Howard bustles in, holding the film of the MRI of my brain in his hands. He does not apologize for the delay. It's almost the opposite. His demeanor is positive. There is no hint of "bad news" as he sits across from us and inserts the MRI film in a fixture designed to display films. He turns it on, turns to us, and begins:

"I do see that you have been diagnosed as having MCI, Sam. You are mildly cognitively impaired. I do have some good news, though. There are no black tangles in your brain."

He turns to his left, scoots his chair closer to the display, and continues: "Look here at the film of your brain. No black tangles, and it is otherwise normal for a fellow your age, with some minor, age-appropriate shrinkage."

Susan and I lean over and squint at the backlit film. I don't see anything that looks like black tangles. We don't know what we are looking for. Dr. Howard stands, picks up the film, and turns off the backlight. He says he has a patient waiting and heads to the door.

Susan and I glance at each other, then I jump up and raise my voice. "Whoa, Dr. Howard, wait! What's going on? What's my prognosis? What's my treatment plan? What road am I on?" I am frustrated and confused.

At the sound of my voice, he stops short and spins around, clearly frustrated and straining to be polite. He doesn't raise his voice. "There is only one road for you, Sam, and that's down. You will only get worse!"

He again starts for the doors, then, unprompted, spins around to face me. He seems to have remembered something and says, "Here, let me give you a prescription for Aricept. It might help." He writes it out on a prescription pad and hands it to me. He seems calm now and says, "You may want to see if you can get into a drug trial of some sort at the University Memory Center in Washington, DC. I know they do drug trials. Now I really have to go, I have patients waiting." He walks out of the room and leaves us alone.

In complete silence, Susan and I sit next to each other in this now-empty room. The out-of-body moment that I am about to experience is familiar to me. I've had them when Susan was delivered "bad news" during her breast cancer journey 15 years before. I am floating above the room, looking down at Susan and myself sitting side-by-side, staring at each other, as if at a portrait of our last moments together. The doctors' words echo in the now-empty room, or maybe just my head: "There is only one road for you, Sam, down. Down! You will only get worse."

Susan and I get up slowly, confused and uncertain, alone in the treatment room. Just the two of us. We struggle to find the way to the front desk. The only person there asks for our name and then tells us that Dr. Howard has left no instructions, and that the office will be in touch IF the doctor wants to see me again.

I don't recall ever feeling so alone in my life. I look around to see if there is anyone else to talk to, or perhaps a brochure or something, or anything to help make sense of what has just happened. Susan tugs at me, and we go down the elevator to our car. Susan takes over.

"Sam, we need to find another doctor. We need a second opinion from someone who can give us a plan for you to get better." I'm not accustomed to feeling so helpless. I need her energy and confidence in that moment.

Over time, I have come to understand two things about this first neurologist encounter.

First, what happened in that room borders on malpractice on multiple levels. Not the least is that one doesn't just take Aricept. Luckily, I didn't fill that prescription. I have learned that with medicines like Aricept, you start with a small dosage and then increase over time, depending on how you react. I also learned that Aricept is typically given in later stages of cognitive decline. The reason is that drugs in this category lose their effectiveness over time. The drug I am on now, not Aricept, will ultimately decrease in its effectiveness. I will eventually be given a different drug, which will also lose effectiveness over time.

The one thing I do know is that it was wrong to prescribe Aricept at all as a first treatment. Also, when Aricept, or any of the typical drugs, including the one that I am now on, are prescribed, there is always a process of slowly increased dosages intermixed with doctor appointments. Dr. Howard didn't know what he was doing. We have since discovered that our Dr. Howard, although a neurologist, was not trained in memory loss issues. As some time passed and I learned more about the disease, and had started to perform my play, *Dementia Man*, I thought I would let him know what had happened to me. I thought it odd that he never reached out after that first appointment. When I looked him up again on the practice website, I saw that he no longer lists memory loss as a field of his practice today.

Second, a diagnosis of Mild Cognitive Impairment does not tell a doctor what is causing the impairment. Yes, he looked at an MRI and saw no "NFTs," neurofibrillary tangles, informally referred to as "tau tangles."

The purpose of the tests, though, are to determine the cause of my MCI. He mentions in our meeting, as he writes the Aricept prescription, that a PET/CT scan with contrast is needed. The PET/CT would provide us with a lot more information. The scan looks for abnormal levels of amyloid proteins, which are primary indicators of Alzheimer's Disease. He does not recommend it because the test is very expensive. Moreover, he doesn't explain at that point why it was important to get such a scan. He just indicates that most people don't get one because of the cost.

As soon as we get home following the appointment, Susan begins the search for a new doctor. She calls her friend Ellen. Ellen and her husband, Paul, belonged to the McLean Racquet and Health Club, and so do we. The four of us are early-morning exercisers. It turns out I had met Paul years before through my work. He was then the president of a prominent Washington, DC-based trade association. He had hired my public affairs company to brief his staff about the then-new "internet" and its emerging use as an advocacy tool. We then bumped into each other at the McLean Racquet Club. I began to understand that he was a true Washington bigshot. Before the trade association work, he had been the private secretary to a president of the United States—a high-profile one. Indeed, his journey is part of American History.

During this time, we learned that a few years before my encounter with Mild Cognitive Impairment, Paul had begun to demonstrate symptoms of cognitive decline. He was eventually diagnosed with Alzheimer's disease. He ultimately moved into a nearby group home, where he lived until he succumbed to the disease.

Susan had been spending time with Ellen, his wife, in various gym classes over the years, so it was a logical phone call after that disastrous visit with my neurologist. "Who was Paul's neurologist, Ellen? Is he good?"

Ellen tells Susan that they liked their neurologist, a Dr. Banks, and that the head of the University Memory Center, Dr. Scott, had recommended him to them. Indeed, Susan and I had attended a lecture by Dr. Scott at Ellen's recommendation. Later in our journey, Dr. Scott will provide me with a second opinion—technically, it was a third opinion—regarding my own decline.

In any case, Susan follows up on the recommendation and calls for an appointment with Dr. Banks's neurology practice. Using Ellen's name as the person who referred us gets us the appointment. Dr. Banks is highly respected and is booked out for the foreseeable future. The first opening we can get is in six weeks.

Yep. "Six more weeks" is still the mantra of our journey with this disease. We recall how Paul slowly disappeared—we could see his decline almost daily as we went to the McLean Racquet Club around seven every morning. Paul would become increasingly unaware of his surroundings. He would sit atop the same stationary bike, peddling, almost in a daze as he stared straight ahead. He would smile and wave, then he stopped waving, though he still smiled—it seemed—and then it was just a blank face and feet turning rotely on the bike. Seeing him decline adds "volume" to the new pressure of my journey in our lives. I don't know how to better describe it than that; the feeling doesn't have a name. Perhaps it's just the augur of lousy news, still in formation, which now occupies ever more space in our lives as a premonition.

It is nearly two years since my earliest, frightful engagements with frustrating cognitive symptoms like driving in circles and going the wrong way down one-way streets, followed by my disappearances into infinite nothingness. When Susan called Ellen for help in finding a neurologist, Paul was already living in a group home. Ellen couldn't take care of him anymore.

By this time, I am getting depressed. I start to think about what to do as I catastrophize the future. I haven't even been diagnosed with Alzheimer's yet. I am trying to digest what Mild Cognitive Impairment—which Dr. Howard said will only get worse—is going to mean to me. Plus, I am still falling in and out of darkness, driving on the wrong side of the road, forgetting appointments, not recognizing people, etc. It is all still there; I am not being treated.

One day, as I begin my 40-minute morning exercise routine at the McLean Racquet Club, I start listening to a podcast with an interview of an author whose husband had early-stage Alzheimer's, which will be my eventual diagnosis. The author is promoting her new book, which I will *not* name here. The book is the story of the journey she and her husband experienced from his diagnosis of early-stage Alzheimer's to his accompanied suicide at Dignitas, a facility in Switzerland. The idea shocks me, and yet as I listen, there is a very brief moment—maybe just a nanosecond—I wonder, "Maybe I should do that too." It sends me into a period of deep personal reflection. Who am I? What are my values? And what should I do?

These are not simple questions, indeed, when we are given the gift—or curse—of knowing we are in our final stages of life. Who am I? What should I do? It will, as you read, take some time for me to figure this out. These are moments when "everything" counts.

Maybe another way to put it is, how do I go into that "good night?"

I reflect deeply on my existential self as I have confronted and moved through this disease. I am telling this story at this point from a retrospective perspective. I know how I am doing "Alzheimer's Disease"—now. I didn't know when it started. It is a bit of a dilemma in my role as author and storyteller. Does setting up the "end" here, spoil the journey? I hope not.

The end, of course, will be later—maybe another five or so years from now, when this 80-year-old man is 85, which would be a long lifetime for anyone these days. Indeed, as you will learn, both my parents passed away in their early 60s.

CHAPTER 3

THE GIFTS OF MY PARENTS

As I get ready to go deeper into my decisions around what to do once diagnosed—how to get ready to go into that good night—I feel compelled to set the baseline of my life and reflect on my growing up. So, allow me to go back, then, to the beginning and tell you a little more about myself: Troublemaker Sam.

It's hard to know when or how it started. The explanation might be as simple as the fact that I was the only boy with four sisters, three of them older than me. Maybe I just needed to cause trouble to get noticed? Except that the typical view is that an only son in a family with four daughters would have been spoiled, because he gets all the attention? Maybe not, if the older sisters are all "stars"—one an "all-star" in tennis, another an acting star, winning a trip to Hollywood. The other sister, closest in age, had special needs. What was left for me to do other than "act out," also known as causing trouble?

It has been a remarkable journey. Really, who would have imagined? I am a kid from El Paso, Texas. I was born there on July 18, 1945. I don't remember anything about that day, nor do I remember if I caused any trouble, though I wouldn't be surprised if I did.

My dad, Marcus Simon, was born in St. Louis, Missouri, and moved with his family to El Paso, Texas, when he was just 5 years old. He graduated from El Paso High School, as did four of his five children, including me. He dropped out of college because of the Great Depression. He eventually became a traveling salesman in the late 1940s, driving around the southwestern desert from El Paso through New Mexico, Arizona, and into Southern California and occasionally into Baja, Mexico. Which meant he was rarely home. The joke was as soon as he returned from a three-, five-, or ten-day trip, people would first ask: "When are you leaving again?" Was my troublemaking because I had no male role model? Or was it to get some attention?

My relationship with my father was always complicated. I felt I kept disappointing him. As a young man, I was skinny and not physically strong. A classic "90-pound weakling" as portrayed in one of the newspaper comics of those days. My dad was a he-man of sorts. He became a wrestler for a period and was part of public wrestling matches across the border from El Paso, in Juarez, Mexico. I think he wanted a son just like him.

It took me some time to come to see my dad's journey as a real-life version of that portrayed in Arthur Miller's famous play, *Death of a Salesman*. First performed in 1949, the play is a classic and typically still required reading in schools. The plot of that book and play seems still to be part of the modern American mindset to the extent that even today when during my performance of *Dementia Man,* when I deliver the line *"My dad was a traveling salesman—think Willie Loman,"* the audience's reaction ranges from giggles to gasps. They know what I'm talking about.

Researching that play again for this book revealed that my memory is not perfect. Like my father, Willy Loman aged poorly and struggled with his work. However, he eventually committed suicide, which my father did not. Well, at least not overtly. I look back and believe my dad thought of himself as a failure. Those were, in fact, his very last words. On his deathbed, having been in and out of a coma for several days, he woke up one morning, sat up, said: "I have been a failure all my life," laid back down, closed his eyes, and took his last breath.

It seemed to me he had done well, selling and making a living for a family of six for many years. At around sixty, Dad had a stroke while he was on the road. It took him at least a year to recover sufficiently to get back on the road. Only a year later, the company was sold. Not long after that, I don't remember how long, in events that echo the storyline of *Death of a Salesman,* my dad walked into the office one day and was told by the new boss he was fired. The new owner explained to my father that he had overpaid for the company, and that it was necessary to fire all but one of the salesmen, effective immediately. My father was fired. No retirement. No health care. No nothing.

This left my family in a financial fix. I was 18 at the time. My dad had to turn to his sister for help. She had married into a wealthy family. Her husband, my dad's brother-in-law, owned and ran a Texaco oil refinery in El Paso. He agreed, at his wife's request, to set my father up to manage a Texaco filling station in town. I was still in college at the time, and I would work some night shifts—for nothing—to give him some time off. To make it worse, one of his other employees stole from him. The filling station was failing, and my father was fired. And that's when he got seriously ill and ended up in that hospital.

My mom worked most of her life, even with a husband who traveled and with five children. We had childcare—a woman from Juarez, Mexico, right across the border from El Paso, would come to our house and live there five days a week, taking care of us while Mom went to work.

Mom. What a lady! She was a flamenco dancer as a young girl. She never graduated from high school. She eventually became a speed typist and a self-taught bookkeeper. The work she went to every day was at a small business in town, and her salary is what kept us afloat during those times Dad got sick. I suspect we got some financial help from my mom's side of the family. It turns out that her dad had been a wealthy businessman in both Florida and Louisiana She had seven siblings!

Her father died in the 1930s, and the remaining sisters supported one another. One of the sisters was a "lawyer"—that is, she had passed the Texas, Louisiana, and Florida bars. She never went to law school, though. She had been working as a legal secretary and learned the law from that position. She was the 16th woman in Florida to be admitted to the Bar, and among the first women in Florida admitted to the Federal Bar. She was among the first women lawyers in three different states: Florida, Louisiana, and Texas! As I learned of the exceptional accomplishments of my Aunt Lena, I saw it as fighting the system, causing trouble. More evidence that I inherited the troublemaker gene from the Alfman family.

Her large family was very loving and supportive of each other, though always seeming to be "outsiders." Mom was a true "Southern Lady" and always wanted me to hang out with the "right people," and to be super successful. And traditional. She always wanted me to be "better." I should hang out with the more "upper-class" folks in the Jewish community. Instead, I played with the regular kids in our neighborhood.

Smoking

Another possible source of my troublemaking energy comes from the journey through smoking, and eventual anger at the world because of how hard it was to stop, even when I urgently needed to end my smoking because of a serious health issue. Smoking was normal, almost universal, as I grew up. Both of my parents were chain smokers. Not only was our home always reeking of cigarette smoke, but the car was also always full of smoke. I suspect driving in a car with the windows up for hours as my dad puffed away was the equivalent of me smoking. He smoked unfiltered Camels, by the way. Like my folks, I became a chain smoker, starting secretly around 13, and openly by 16.

What's a chain smoker? Someone who will smoke continuously. As soon as one cigarette is done, they take out another one and light it up. They may smoke twenty to forty to maybe even sixty cigarettes a day. That's about three packs or more, since there are twenty cigarettes in a pack. Of course, this was all before the Surgeon General said smoking was not good for people. I wonder now to what extent my heavy smoking contributed to my own health issues—the period in which I had cluster vascular migraines forty years ago, and now potentially a factor in my neurocognitive decline. The research I have done suggests smoking and migraines can increase the risk of Alzheimer's by 30 percent above the average person.

My first puff on a cigarette was on one of several traveling salesman trips with my father. Every year, there was a "market" event at The Adams, a hotel in Phoenix, Arizona, and my dad and one of the other salesmen from the same company would host a "sample room." The son of Dad's colleague came on this trip. I think we were both 13 at the time. We snuck away one day by walking out onto the fire escape platform just outside a window on the fifth floor of the hotel. It was at the end of a long hallway, so no one would see us. That is where we each had our first puff on a cigarette. I remember feeling dizzy and sick to my stomach and thinking I didn't want to do it again. And yet I did. Again and again for 25 years.

I remember the moment I started smoking in front of my parents. I was 16 years old and had been smoking behind their backs for two years or so. I was already hooked. Then came the time that my family was going to visit my oldest sister, Marion, who was living in Washington, DC. She was 25, I was 16. We would drive from El Paso to Washington, DC, and back.

The trip was three days long, and with Mom, Dad, and two sisters, the car was packed. A half day into the trip, I had to do something, so I confessed I was smoking. I found out everyone knew I was smoking. Despite my young age, they reluctantly said yes to my request—demand—that I be allowed to smoke. I can still remember the conversation among the three adults: "How can we tell him 'No' when all of us smoke?"

By the time I was in college, two years later, I had become a chain smoker. I had already met Susan, and we were in a serious relationship. One night, we were studying together in my parents' home where I lived. We had opened a card table in the living room and were sitting together, I with an ashtray full of cigarette butts. I decided to persuade Susan to smoke, too. She had just lit the cigarette I had given her and was puffing on it, but not inhaling it. I was trying to teach her to inhale when my mother walked into the room, cigarette in hand.

"Sam, don't teach her to smoke, it's not healthy," Mom announces, cigarette in her hand. She then turns and puffs on her cigarette as she leaves.

I finally stopped smoking in 1978, 17 years after starting.

Conquering my addiction to nicotine and stopping smoking was the hardest thing I ever had to do in my life. Still, 46 years later, I believe nothing has been more difficult. Not even coming to terms with my Alzheimer's! As I went through this process, I developed a sense of outrage and anger against the tobacco industry and the government for not outlawing cigarettes.

I needed to stop smoking around 1976, after the onset of the previously mentioned cluster vascular migraine headaches. Of course, I didn't know what they were at the time, only that periodically, it felt like someone was pressing a super-hot iron into the right side of my brain. That was the first time I saw a neurologist—they treated such headaches. The experience was fine, that is until the neurologist said he couldn't continue treating me unless I stopped smoking. Of course, he was correct because everything else he had tried had not stopped the headaches, and his next course of treatment involved a drug that had significant side effects.

Even with this incentive—ending the worst pain known to humans—it took some time before I could finally figure out how to stop. I tried and tried, and the damage to my self-image was significant. It reminded me of those early-in-life low self-esteem years. I would invest my entire ego into the project. *I am a sentient being capable of doing this because I need to for me and my family,* I would tell myself. And then I failed and failed. I finally signed up for a Smoke Enders program, and it worked. I believe it worked because by that time, I had literally "given up"—I signed up for the program because someone told me it had worked for them.

The afternoon of the first class in a large hotel meeting room in downtown Washington, DC, I walked through the door, positive this too would NOT work for me. Looking back years later, I understood that, in some weird way, that attitude helped me quit. The mindset was a form of surrender; if it was not going to work, I didn't need to resist or try too hard. Most important to my success, I suspect, was that the first thing the teacher said that day, standing up on a podium in front of about 40 students, was "light 'em up." Life was good.

I wonder if my heavy smoking, and perhaps even those migraines, had anything to do with developing Alzheimer's. I just looked that up, and there does seem to be "some evidence" that migraines and "dementia" are related. Yes, having smoked increases the risk of Alzheimer's by about 1.8 percent compared to non-smokers.

The Gift of a Genetic Risk

In addition to the increased health risks from smoking, I have a genetic risk associated with Alzheimer's. Early on in my Alzheimer's journey, I learned that there is a gene—it is called APOE. It has three variations, and as I understand, an ApoE2 means you are less likely to develop Alzheimer's. ApoE3 is "neutral" according to NIH, and it means your risk is average or typical. Finally, there is an ApoE4 version that is associated with an increased risk of Alzheimer's disease. Almost all people with Alzheimer's disease have one or two ApoE4 genes. We inherit our genes from either or both parents. As an aside, a 2024 study has suggested that people with two instances of ApoE4, meaning that both parents have the gene, should be treated as if they already have Alzheimer's as they grow up. People, like me, with one instance of an ApoE4 gene are two to three times more likely to have Alzheimer's, and those with two instances of the ApoE4 gene are 8 to 12 times more likely to have Alzheimer's than the average.

My ApoE4 gene, I believe, is inherited from my paternal grandmother's family. That is my grandmother on my father's side. My father's mother, Grandma Simon, was born Clara Blonder. I have been in touch with the current generation of Blonders. There is and has been, according to them, a lot of Alzheimer's disease in their extended family. A number of the current generation have been tested, and several have an instance of ApoE4. I also learned that Alzheimer's has been in several earlier generations of that family line. It is always possible that there are other sides of the family with ApoE4, I just don't know for sure.

Alzheimer's risks from my mother's side could exist because genes can skip a generation. So far, though, I can find no one from my mother's side of the family with Alzheimer's. However, my Aunt Julia, my mother's sister, and my sister, Harriet, both had significantly low intellectual functioning. I hesitate to use the word "cognitive" because we never used that term in talking about them, nor the word "dementia." Although late in life, my Aunt Lena, who lived until her mid-80s, became significantly impaired, she was never diagnosed with Alzheimer's. I mentioned previously, she was a notable woman: The sixteenth woman to be licensed to practice law in Florida, despite never going to law school. She was also one of the earliest women to be admitted to the bar and be licensed to practice in Louisiana, Texas, and the Federal Bar in Florida.

The possibility of an Alzheimer's diagnosis was never on my radar screen. The truth is that over a decade ago, when I subscribed to 23andMe to find relatives and sent a specimen, their report told me that I had an instance of the ApoE4 and was thus at "slightly higher risk" for Alzheimer's. It meant nothing to me at that time. Now, with a diagnosis and the knowledge that the disease is often hereditary, I wish I had paid closer attention back then. Yes, now I know—or at least I believe—that my diagnosis of Alzheimer's Disease is one of those "gifts of my family."

CHAPTER 4

EXISTENTIAL TRAINING

So now, Sam Simon, the son of Marcus and Frieda, the former heavy smoker, the man whose genetic make-up perhaps made this existential moment inevitable, is sitting down, trying to figure out if he should go to Switzerland and kill himself.

That "nanosecond" of wondering—*Should I go to Switzerland and commit suicide?*—takes me into a deep dive on what to do next. At that moment, I don't feel depressed; I am just confused, confronting a whole new life circumstance. I don't know what I should do. I have had other medical issues. I have been hospitalized only twice. First, because I had a pulmonary embolism. Yes, a blood clot in my lung. I was under the watchful eye of a pulmonary specialist for more than a decade, and the conclusion was that it was simply the result of traveling on airplanes and not moving around enough.

The other long-term issue for me was prostatitis. I have had multiple biopsies, and about ten years ago, my urologist was sure I had prostate cancer. I had surgery to reduce the size of the prostate to reduce the risk of cancer. In January 2025, that changed. Bloody urine and an MRI of the prostate revealed the presence of cancer. I am now in the "watchful waiting" process. Prostate cancer is sort of an "old man's" disease. According to the American Cancer Society, approximately 80 percent of men over the age of 80 have prostate cancer. It's no fun either, though not as serious as Alzheimer's.

Only at this moment, newly diagnosed with Alzheimer's, working out on the elliptical machine, and hearing a woman interviewed saying that she supported her husband in getting to Switzerland to kill himself, does it occur to me I should consider ending my life. As you will read, I am very human and have lived a life of ups and downs. Yet, it never occurred to me that my life was not worth living. Even now, with Alzheimer's and cancer, it is not a thought. Indeed, the more I hear about and read about the campaigns in support of end-of-life suicide, the more I can't imagine making that choice.

Oddly, before I was thirty, I had spent numerous moments being around death. Indeed, I sometimes think of myself as an "existential journeyman." I didn't always describe myself that way. It is a more recent interpretation of my life history. Once, I hosted a small meeting of new acquaintances—a few rabbis, ministers, and me. We were all going to be part of a new project I was leading, and we decided to spend a couple of hours getting to know each other better. We started with an introductory roundtable, where we each gave a brief description of ourselves. I said: "I am an existential dancer." By that, I was adapting the phrase from the first book I had written about nearly losing my wife, then of 34 years, to breast cancer, and referred to that experience as "the actual dance." The end of life ritual, an ecstatic moment with Susan and me in the center of a ballroom that floated in a liminal space, in which we were surrounded by everyone we ever met, ever knew, even generations before us, and maybe yet to come, as we danced to the music of our hearts, and Susan would take her last breath, and leave my arms.

Today, I would have introduced myself by saying, "I am an existential troublemaker."

Who and what am I, or perhaps "are we" in this world? How long will we live? What is our purpose, and what should be accomplished? These are, for me, existential questions. It had never occurred to me to use the word "existential" much, if at all, in my life, notwithstanding that I have spent significant real-world time engaged with just these matters. Not until I was diagnosed with a terminal disease, that is.

I remember noticing in my early forties and fifties how very few of my friends had ever experienced the loss of a loved one. Usually, I would hear of their grief over the loss of a grandparent. By then, I had gone through two sets of grandparents, my parents, a sibling, my wife's parents, cousins, and dear friends. Indeed, I had already been in the room while someone took their last breath.

My first memory of death was when I was five years old. It was a Sunday morning, and I was jarred awake by a commotion in the house.

Five-year-old Sam, in his pajamas, waddles out of his bedroom into a hallway that runs the length of the back of the house to a door that opens into a stairwell down to the driveway of our house. "The back door." It was a single-level house, except that the back of the property was lower than the front. So, to keep the house "level," as the property sloped down, there was an ever-larger crawl space underneath the house, and the back of the house required a stairway, off to the side, to get out the back. That morning, my parents and maybe an older sister or two were leaving very early out that back door of our house.

"What's going on?" I remember yelling.

"Grandpa died," someone shouted.

My father's father, Sidney Simon, married to Clara Blonder, was one of 11 children of my great-grandfather, Marcus Simon. It is a Jewish tradition to always name a child after an ancestor, never a living relative. Thus, my father was named after my great-grandfather, Marcus Simon. My Dad's grandfather, Marcus Simon, had passed before my dad was born. In that same vein, our son is named after my father, his grandfather, who passed before he was born. Thus, our son is Marcus Simon.

I remember being told that I, 5-year-old Sammy, was too young to go to the funeral of my grandfather, Sidney Simon.

My next memory of death is of my grandmother on my mother's side. Grandma Alfman, to me. Earnestine

Alfman was her name. Of all my ancestors, she lived the longest. She died at 88 years old. The burial was followed by a "mourners' meal" at the bereaved family's home—a tradition in most Jewish families. That meant our house. My parents had decided that I was still too young to be allowed to go to the funeral; I was 9 years old at the time. I was also asked to stay in my bedroom during this event at our house.

As I lie on the bed reading or something, I can overhear the chattering noise of everyone in the living room area. I feel excluded and quite sorry for myself. Suddenly, my mother barges into the room. She is sobbing. I think it is the first time I ever experienced my mother crying. She doesn't even acknowledge me as she enters the room and heads straight to a closet opposite my bed. She tries to reach something up in the closet but can't, comes out to grab a small stand, re-enters the closet, and steps on the stand to reach the very top to take something down. Yes, I can picture that moment today, 2025, as if it were yesterday—actually, it was the afternoon of May 17, 1954.

"Why are you crying?" I ask as she turns to leave and rejoin the others. She swirls toward me and barks, "You would cry too if your mother died." It totally confuses me. She is my mother! What is she talking about?

With time, I frequently found myself in death's presence—my grandparents, my parents, Susan's parents. Most of these have occurred before Susan and I were 30 years old. My sister Harriet was just two years older than me and passed in her early thirties from cancer.

In terms of my mother, I was in the room with her as she took her last breath, and that was in my late 20s. The moment in the hospital with her as she died was perhaps the most consequential moment in my spiritual life. Or, arguably, my life.

Two nurses and I are alone in her hospital room. Our family has agreed to suspend medical care; there isn't even a heart monitor. Medical directives were not widely used in 1967; instead, there were informal agreements between families and doctors. Mom had lost cognitive awareness weeks before; her breast cancer had metastasized to her brain, she didn't recognize any of us, and just lay in bed, occasionally mumbling unintelligibly.

No machine starts to buzz loudly when her heart stops—just us three, two nurses and me, around sunset, waiting. My older sister, Evelyn, was supposed to join me, but she was having issues at home that delayed her departure. I was alone in the room when the two nurses enter. They look at my mother, they look at me. Each nurse from opposite sides of the bed takes a wrist, feels for a pulse, glance at each other, nod, turn towards me, and say, "She's gone."

At that instant, my eyes start to tear up, and I begin to turn toward my left, away from the dead body on the bed, when I experience my first truly "existential moment." A swirling tuft of white cloud swooshes from my mother, almost as if arising from her body, slows slightly as it moves across from me, as if to say goodbye, and then swishes out of the room—all done at what feels like the speed of light.

I understood then and still believe today that the "tuft of white cloud" was her soul exiting this world.

The next existential journey is when Susan is diagnosed with stage-3, triple-negative breast cancer, the same illness that took her mother and my mother. One day, not long after Susan's double mastectomy, the doctors pull me aside to tell me to "get ready." They do not expect her to survive. My experience is going to be one of anticipatory grief—I start the grieving process in advance of her actual, anticipated death. She survives, and nearly ten years later, I end up writing a play and book about that experience, *The Actual Dance: Love's Ultimate Journey Through Breast Cancer.*

And there is more. In my 60s, I hold the medical power of attorney for my dear friend, Rabbi Richard Sternberger, of blessed memory. He had been the adjunct rabbi of our temple for many, many years. We shared a passion for social justice. Indeed, he had been a national social justice leader in the Reform Jewish movement during his career, while I was at the same time being a high-visibility public advocate working with Ralph Nader. In his retirement, he had a bad fall, which caused a severe brain bleed. I ended up being the person to decide if the doctors should withhold treatment. I was also in the room with him when he took his last breath. Another existential moment.

Even though I have spent much of my time engaged in existential moments—life and death—I had, of course, never been diagnosed with a terminal illness until now. Never before have I had to face my mortality.

In retrospect, I think my inner longing had always been to be a rabbi, a spiritual caregiver. I remember Rabbi Fierman, my growing-up rabbi. Our family was close to him, and he wrote about our family in several of his books. I remember admiring him during my late teens and early 20s. All these years later, it feels that I admired him most for giving comfort, teaching, and helping people.

So here I am, a rabbi wannabe, experiencing other people's grief, being with others as they go through their end-of-life journey. Then my own time, with the love of my life, my soul mate, the "other half of my whole," Susan, traveling with her as we go up to the edge of the abyss. I am there to hold her hand; we give each other strength. She is braver than I, and of course, we can't imagine that our roles will eventually be reversed. Now, she is always there for me as I approach that abyss.

Yet, at that moment early in this journey, as I exercised on the elliptical machine, the question suddenly became: "What should I do?" I heard it in my ear that day—that I was going to become a "lesser and lesser person." Would I unfairly impose that "longest day"—what many have come to call the Alzheimer's disease journey—onto Susan?

Despite my history of being with others as they approached their death, and indeed with them in that moment, I don't think I was yet equipped to answer that question. I only remember that emotion, the feeling of anger, "No! I have more to do."

CHAPTER 5

BECOMING A TROUBLEMAKER

As I write this book, I've just finished my 80th year, diagnosed with a terminal disease. Susan and I are not a portrait of the stereotypical folks in their 70s and 80s living in an "old age home"—we call them senior living communities today. The typical picture is of people with walkers and canes playing bridge and watching TV all day long. Some sewing or knitting. Not us.

Somehow, with Susan's support, I am out there in the world, trying to swim against the tide of this disease, shaking things up, and trying to be part of—even a leader of—a new movement to reimagine the journey of cognitive decline. While writing this, I was mentioned in a guest editorial comment in the New York Times as part of that movement.

Yes, even as I enter my final stage of life, I do not go gently. As the title of one of the classic books in the dementia field declares, I am living a life, screaming: "I AM STILL HERE." Yes, as I am going away, I am causing trouble.

I sometimes wonder where my tendency to cause trouble originated. The fact is that from the time I was a kid to my first real job—I was a form of a troublemaker.

As a young man, it drove my parents crazy.

My mom, born Frieda Alfman, always seemed very different than my dad. Her gift to me, I think, is the troublemaker gene. I have not heard of a gene that creates troublemakers, and I would not be surprised if it is discovered one day. There is a distinct energy I feel, an urge, which enables me to see something as unfair or wrong, and to act to change. Of course, as a young kid, it was seen more as me just acting out.

My mother's father, Harry Alfman, and mother, Ernestine Alfman, nee Klonover, were from Poland. Harry, who I understand was a stowaway on a ship when he was just 19 years old—seems like troublemaking—arrived in Montgomery, Alabama, and then moved to Pensacola, Florida. He did very well as a businessman. He appeared, too, to have somehow connected to the family that later founded Macy's Department Store.

He relocated his growing family to New Orleans in 1907, taking his then-born daughter, Frieda, my mother, born in Pensacola before the move. The story behind that move is the most significant indication that he was a troublemaker.

It wasn't until I was in my sixties that I learned about Harry Alfman's life. He was a small business owner in both Pensacola, Florida, and New Orleans. Amazingly, he secured a patent for an umbrella part, which might have generated some of his apparent wealth. The family lore has been that he was poor, and that does not seem to be true. He owned a small business that performed metal work for ships and provided construction services to the community.

In 1906, a major hurricane, described as the worst in 170 years, hit the Gulf Coast of Florida, including Pensacola. Among the damage it caused was the destruction of the roof of Pensacola's City Hall. The city contracted with Harry Alfman's business to install a new roof. The city believed he had cheated them by billing more for workers' wages than he paid the workers. So, they charged him with fraud and issued a warrant for his arrest. He promptly fled to Tennessee. I can't imagine how that happened, since he had six young children and a wife. The Pensacola sheriff obtained an extradition order from a court and brought him back for trial. The story made headlines in the local newspapers, which is how I learned all these details. It turned out that the city had one prosecutor, and my grandfather had three defense lawyers and 42 character witnesses. He was acquitted. Maybe I take after my grandfather Alfman!

After that incident, Harry moved his family to New Orleans. As mentioned, my mother, Frieda Alfman, was born in the middle of this uproar. I wonder if her father was even home when she was born or had been hiding in Tennessee by then. I do know that they had already sold their Pensacola home and were ready to move to New Orleans before the trial.

My mother had six sisters and one brother. The brother was named Sam Alfman. Sam developed tuberculosis, commonly referred to as TB, while they were in New Orleans. In that era, there was no cure. The only option was to move to a higher elevation. For them, that was El Paso, Texas, 3,700 feet above sea level. El Paso is divided by Mt. Franklin, the last of the Rocky Mountains. Technically, which I learned while writing this book, it is called North Franklin Mountain. The last of the Franklin Mountain Range, it is the tail end of the Rocky Mountains, which start in Colorado, come through New Mexico, and end in the center of El Paso, Texas. North Franklin Mountain (we never called it that) has an altitude of 7,192 feet. Growing up, and until now, I knew it only as Mount Franklin. We lived on a street—the exact address was 1149 Galloway—which dead-ended at the base of a smaller mountain called "Crazycat." Crazycat was a small mountain compared to Mt Franklin. It is where, as a kid, I, with the other kids in the neighborhood, would climb and play.

The Alfman family's move to El Paso was permanent. When they arrived, Harry Alfman and his seven children, including Sam Alfman, were greeted by the El Paso rabbi, Martin Zelonka. The only rabbi in El Paso at the time, he was the rabbi of Temple Mt. Sinai, which is still the reform synagogue in El Paso. Sam was hired to work as the secretary to the rabbi for about a year before passing away. The connection to the rabbi and the way the family was embraced in El Paso has always been for me an indication that the Alfmans were a well-known and respected family.

Like the Alfmans, I, too, have been very active both in our local and the national Reform Jewish community. I have served as president of our temple in Falls Church,

Virginia, and I served on the Board of Advisors to Hebrew Union College, the national Reform Jewish Seminary. As of the time of this book, I am emeritus to that Board, and I am on the Board of Visitors to the Debbi Friedman School of Sacred Music.

I never knew Sam, nor Harry Alfman. I do remember my grandmother, his wife, Ernestine Alfman, nee Klonover. She lived in our house for a few years and passed when I was 9 years old. I also remember many of the other Alfman girls, including my mother, Frieda, her sisters, Sarah, Johanna, Etta, and Lena. I did not know Rose. My mother, of course, was born Frieda Alfman. She married my dad, Marcus Simon. I don't know why, but she always used her maiden name as her middle name. "Frieda Alfman Simon." Our family lived on the West Side of the mountain, a five-minute walk to Crazycat, in the neighborhood known as Kern Place.

My parents met in El Paso and had five children. Like the Alfman side of the family, I was the only boy. Three sisters were older than me: Marion, nine years older, Evelyn, seven years older, and Harriet, two years older. Then, one younger, Sylvia Sue, five years younger. Evelyn and Sue are still around. Harriet passed away first, from cancer, when she was just 32. Marion, the oldest, lived to 86.

So here is the picture: Dad, the traveling salesman, is on the road most of the time. My mom, four sisters, and I are at home together without him. My main memory from those days was the 6:01 p.m. Sunday telephone calls. Long-distance rates fell sharply on Sundays after 6 p.m. You dial zero, get the operator, give them the number of the hotel where to call, we get connected, then everyone gets five minutes with Dad. I remember once, when he had changed hotels, we asked the operator to call around the hotels in whatever city it was to find him. They did that!

I think being the only boy in that household prompted me to start causing trouble back then. In retrospect, what else could I do? I know, the stereotype of the situation is that I would have been a spoiled brat. Only boy, four sisters. Perhaps it could have been that, but Dad was never around. So, I didn't have a male model, and Mom was swamped. She had to work and raise five children. We had a full-time "maid." This was not unusual in El Paso at that time. The maid, a citizen of Juarez, Mexico, across the Rio Grande from El Paso, lived in our house during the week, and she spoke mainly Spanish. I'm told I spoke Spanish before I spoke English.

It is hard to remember what exactly came first. I never heard any talk of my being a difficult birth—the fourth child—though I suspect I might have been. Or maybe my troublemaking didn't start until I was two years old and fell on the "floor furnace" one day. That is how we heated the home back then. A floor furnace was basically a stove built into the floor, with gas burners creating heat that rose through a metal grate. Apparently, or so I am told, I fell on the hot grate when I was 2, and burned the inside of my right leg on the grill. A grill-like scar developed on my leg that did not disappear until I was 30. I don't remember the moment, just that I kept being reminded of the cause of that scar and how much of a big deal it was at the time it happened.

Even in grade school, I somehow found a way to cause trouble. My recollection of my grade school time was of me as an outsider—skinny, with few friends, and occasionally bullied. I think it was around the time I was in first grade that trouble started. Yes, in first grade, I had a "girlfriend." Her name was Cathy Harper, yes, I remember. Don't ask. We were, by that time, gender curious. We were both students at Mesita Elementary in El Paso.

We lived near Mesita School, and even as a first grader, I would walk the 0.6 of a mile to school every day. Cathy, though, lived farther away and rode a city bus to school every day. Cathy and I would hang out together during recess and at other times. Even sneaking off to be alone with each other, sometimes into a bathroom. We had a sense of being boyfriend and girlfriend. Really!

Cathy asked me if I wanted to go home with her one day. I say sure, but I don't have the money for a "bus ticket"—5 cents each. She says to come anyway, and she somehow persuades the bus driver to accept a torn-in-half ticket—half for her and half for me. I don't think of asking how I will get home. I am just feeling special. My first date.

I don't know what I am expecting. At least meeting her parents and maybe having an afternoon snack. We get off the bus on Stanton Street, one of the major north-south streets, down a big hill from Kern Place to near downtown El Paso. At the time, I was familiar with the area, and I followed her. We walk across the street; she points out her home, the fourth house on the left side, halfway down the block where we are standing: "See, that's my house." Then she says goodbye.

I am stuck. I have no money to take the bus back, so I walk home. It takes about an hour or so. Typically, I am home around noon. Today I return around 2 p.m. As I approach the house, I notice a police car parked in front. Yes, my parents have already called the police and reported me missing. Boy, am I in trouble.

I don't remember much about my oldest sister, Marion, as I was growing up. Usually, the table talk was about her success as a tennis player. She was in a statewide tournament once. I don't remember if she won that one. By the time I was nine, she had already left the house to attend the University of Texas in Austin. I think she and I share the troublemaker gene. I'll talk more about that later.

Evelyn, the second-oldest sister, is seven years older than I am. The big blow-up with her was when she was heading off to the High School prom night—Queen of the Prom—and I whacked her on the back with an open hand, above the dress line, leaving a bright red hand mark. Boy, was I in trouble then.

Over the years, things didn't change much. I wonder if all this was the result of one boy with four sisters trying to get some attention. I especially got in trouble over political stuff. I was, for some reason, already a liberal Democrat. My parents were big FDR fans since the Great Depression had greatly impacted them and their families, and FDR's New Deal meant a lot to them financially.

On the other hand, my mother, born in Pensacola, Florida, and raised in New Orleans, Louisiana, was not a role model for politically progressive outrage. Just the opposite. She was the model of a proper, deeply "Southern Lady." For her, there were "the right kind of people" and "the wrong kind of people." She didn't want us, the Simon kids, to be involved with the de la Garza kids, the Mexican American family living down the street. They had one boy, Henry, and whenever Mom caught me playing with him outside in the front yard or on the street corner, she called me into the house. "He is not the right kind of person." That, too, got me in a tizzy. Even now, all these years later, I don't like to think of the racist undertones of those experiences.

A side note: it turns out that Henry eventually married a nice Jewish girl. He converted to Judaism. They live in Houston, Susan's hometown, and Susan and I periodically see them when we visit Susan's family. My mom would now approve!

Speaking of Henry, he was involved in the first instance in which I had my name in the El Paso newspaper (other than my birth announcement). I believe this was around October 1957, shortly after the Soviet Union launched Sputnik. It was supposed to fly over El Paso one very cloudy night, and Henry and I were outside trying to spot it. We noticed a star-like object moving in the sky between clusters of clouds. We were positive it was Sputnik. I don't remember how or where, only that we were able to contact the local newspaper to report what we saw. Remember there were only plain old dial-up phones back then. In any case, that was considered news back then. The story was printed on the front page. In retrospect, I'm pretty sure it was the clouds that were moving, and the bright star just seemed to move relative to them.

It did not take me much longer to cause enough trouble to get in the newspapers again: two years, 1959.

The 1950s, especially the late 1950s, were unsettled times. It was the beginning of the civil rights movement in the United States. The Simon family finally got a black-and-white television in our home around 1955 or '56. I remember watching as schools in the South were being integrated following the Brown vs Board of Education Supreme Court decision and the resistance to that integration. I saw very similar treatment by the powerful people in El Paso of the Chicanos (the word that was used to describe the Mexican American kids).

Around this time, El Paso, a border town, was experiencing a significant amount of crime in and around the parts of town nearest the border crossing—the entry point to the US. The El Paso City Council's response was to enact an 11 p.m. curfew for kids 17 and younger. The goal, they said, was to reduce vandalism and teen crime.

It was 1959, I was just 14 years old, and I was outraged by the curfew. It is supposed to apply to everyone, but I see through that ruse. The curfew is only enforced in the mainly Hispanic-populated neighborhoods. No one in our middle-class neighborhood ever gets hassled. It riles me up, and I decide to do something about it.

I do some research. I don't remember exactly how I did the research; it must have been in the library. No internet back then. I learn that the newly elected governor of New York, Nelson Rockefeller, thinks such curfews are unconstitutional. So, one day, I march down to a city council meeting. I'm two years away from getting a driver's license, so I take the "Mesita" bus to Plaza Park and then walk to the courthouse. I don't tell my parents about my plan.

I don't remember what I wore. I had a coat and tie from my Bar Mitzvah when I was 13. I do remember the floor-to-ceiling doors composed of elegant mahogany wood at the entry to the City Council Chambers. I had never been there before. I slowly push open one of these giant doors and walk timidly into the room. It is set almost like a courtroom, with audience seats separated by a short railing barrier with a gate into the area where the councilmen sit around a long table. I expected a room full of people and walked instead into an almost empty space, with maybe one or two other visitors.

At the end of their regular agenda, the chairman of the City Council asks if any of the citizens—me and one other person—have any other business. With my stomach in my throat, I raise my hand and walk through the small gate separating the Council table from the seats for citizens. Then, I lecture them on the evils of the curfew. I had done my homework. I tell them that even Nelson Rockefeller believed curfews were unconstitutional. I give them hell for discriminating against the Chicano (Hispanic) kids since the curfew was only enforced in their neighborhoods, not where I lived. They listened politely and then told me, 14-year-old Sam Simon, "Wait until you have teenage kids, young man, then you will understand." They thanked me for coming, asked if anyone else wanted to speak, and when nobody did, adjourned the meeting.

I think back to the Sam Simon of 1959 and then look at Sam Simon of me now, and, yes, it seems to me that the emotional-justice hot button is genetic or inherent. It is a specific emotion that I still experience 65 years later: The moment when every sinew of my body tightens, I have an urgent sense of the need to act, challenge the established order, or speak out. It has directed my life story. I wonder now if it isn't working to help me defy the odds, for a while, of this Alzheimer's diagnosis.

I hadn't noticed the reporter in the room at the City Council meeting; I suppose there is always a reporter present at public city council meetings. The next day, my "rant" was a headline in the morning newspaper. That is how my parents found out what I had done. Boy, was I in trouble, especially with my mother.

My voice for justice was probably set back when I was 14. I was a freshman in high school, El Paso High. My Dad and three older sisters had been students there. El Paso High was a family tradition.

My next troublemaking event is just one year later, when I am a sophomore. I was taking an introductory course in civics. I don't remember the exact title of the course, although I recall the teacher, Ms. Reid, and her appearance. Heavy-set with bright, dyed red hair. Glasses. Always looking disheveled. She was as politically conservative as you can get. One day, Ms. Reid was teaching about the New Deal, specifically about government-funded projects, such as the creation of the Tennessee Valley Authority, which brought electricity to rural areas. According to her, this government-owned and operated electricity system was socialism to its core. Evil! So, she ranted in the class. I argued and argued with her during class. One day, she became so angry with me that she accused me of being disrespectful and kicked me out of class. The vice-principal, Mr. Estes, paddled me and sent me home for two days.

The feedback from my friends was positive. Indeed, my public classroom fight made me a bit of a cult hero. I suspect that was a significant step in my troublemaking journey. I kept speaking out.

The next event was at the end of my junior year. I was in the El Paso High School marching band; I played the tuba. That meant I was at all the high school football games. I noticed that only girls were cheerleaders. I don't know why that bothered me. It did, though, enough for me to do something radical. At El Paso High, cheerleaders were elected, and I decided to run for cheerleader. Yes, an absurd idea; I had no natural physical rhythm or dance talents.

No boy had ever run for cheerleader until I did. When I announced my candidacy, a classmate, Lorenzo Gonzales, decided to run as well. The competition involved an all-school assembly, with those competing going on stage and performing some scripted cheers. The students in the assembly then selected the cheerleader through voice and clapping. Even though I was playing tennis then and almost made the varsity tennis team, the truth is that I was (and still am) a bit of a klutz (Yiddish for clumsy person) and have no sense of rhythm. I lost. Lorenzo won. All the rest were girls. I still take credit for integrating males into the school cheerleading squad, which has long since become the norm.

I think by my senior year in high school, my future was predetermined; I just did not realize it. The American political scene was heating up. Texas, at the time, was mainly a Democratic state, with Lyndon Johnson and Ralph Yarborough being the US senators. John Connally was the Governor and was a Democrat at the time! All my family were Democrats.

I had an interest in politics, and even predicted, in my senior year, that I would be a State legislator one day. (I wrote that prediction in the *Spur,* the high school yearbook, of my friend (and still friend) Richard (Dick) Eger. Dick still reminds me of my "failure" to achieve that goal, even though my son is a Virginia state legislator.

I recall a sense of constant unease about what was happening in the world. Political differences were growing brighter, and it would be later in that year that President Kennedy would be assassinated. One of the significant national developments of that time was the emergence of a far-right group called the John Birch Society. When a chapter was formed in El Paso, Texas, the newspaper provided it with extensive local coverage.

My troublemaker genes lit up. I wanted to expose them. I planned to "join" them, write a paper about the experience and the Society for my high school senior thesis, and then submit it to the local newspaper.

First, though, I thought it was important to protect myself. I didn't know for sure what I was going to do in life, and whatever it was, having been a member of what most people saw as an extremist, radical group might be a problem. My parents agreed. There was a lawyer that my family knew, Mr. Frank Merskey. I made an appointment to ask for his advice. He was fascinated by the project and agreed with the need for caution. He prepared an affidavit for me and witnessed it, which contained details about my project and stated that I did not adhere to their agenda. I could produce the affidavit if my membership in the Society ever came up in my life.

Mr. Mersky also suggested I consider a career in law. I eventually did, and it allowed me to take my troublemaking to a whole new level. I ended up attending just one John Birch Society meeting as a 17-year-old, during which the members largely ignored me. I don't remember much else, and I never wrote the paper. I did, however, for some unknown reason, keep my membership card and carried it in my wallet. More later ... about that card.

It seems that at this point in my life, something happens almost every year, even as I graduate from high school. At the start of this chapter, I mentioned that my grandfather, Harry Alfman, my mother's dad, may be the genetic source of my troublemaker instincts, was charged with criminal fraud. Like him, I too would have a run-in with the law. I even spent a few hours sitting behind bars!

It is a week after high school graduation in 1963. My friend Gary and I celebrated our graduation by using a fake ID to buy some beer. In those days in El Paso, you had to be 21 to drink beer. We drove to one of those eat-in-your-car restaurants called The Oasis on the opposite side of town from where we lived. In our minds, it was to avoid being seen and getting in trouble.

Sitting in the car, we toasted each other, took a swig of our beer, when a car that had just passed stopped short, backed up, and stopped in front of us. Blocking in case we tried to leave. Two agents of the Texas Liquor Control Board get out, approach our car, and ask for our ID. Seeing that we are only 17, they tell us we're under arrest and to follow them to a local Justice of the Peace. The Justice of the Peace, it turns out, lives in a trailer park. When the agents knock on his door around 11 p.m., he answers dressed in a night robe. After holding a brief "trial," he fines us each $20 and $29.95 in court costs. Well, we have $50 between us. We flip a coin to see who gets to have their fine paid. I lose. So, the agents drive me down to the El Paso city jail, about fifteen miles away. I am processed into the "jail," though they let me stay in the holding cell next to the main desk, as long as my fine gets paid in the next two hours. Just in time, two hours later, my friend Gary was able to scrape up another $50. I don't tell my parents anything about this until I'm in my late 20s.

I was reminded of this again in my 60s when Susan and I applied for our Global Entry cards. I did not list that incident on my application, thinking my record as a minor would have been erased. When we returned to pick them up, the border control agent began to hand me my Global Entry card, then pulled it back abruptly. In a humorous tone, said, "Wait, did you forget to tell us something happened when you were 18 years old?"

After he could no longer hold back a grin, he handed my Global Entry card to me.

Another mystery for me now, looking back to that time, is precisely how it happened that I would then spend the rest of the summer of 1963, before starting college at Texas Western in El Paso, living with my oldest sister, Marion, in Washington, DC.

Marion, nine years older than me, was my model for troublemaking, my secret advisor whenever I got in real trouble with my parents. Marion graduated from college before I started high school. Her first job was to work for the National Student Association, a controversial group made up of college student leaders, and often labeled as a communist front, which was eventually revealed to be a CIA-infiltrated organization. She had recently moved from Philadelphia to Washington, DC.

I wanted to get away from home. I was interested in and applied to Antioch College, which was considered a very liberal institution. I don't think I fully understood then that my parents didn't have the money. Additionally, my high school grade average was a C-, which was not high enough to gain admission to Antioch. My parents proposed that I stay in El Paso for at least one year, get my grade point average up, and then see if I could get into the University of Texas in Austin. That is what my sister Marion had done.

I wasn't happy. I was beyond eager to leave home after high school, so my parents came up with the idea for me to spend the summer in Washington, DC, between high school graduation and starting college. I would stay with Marion in her Washington, DC, apartment. While our family trip to Washington, DC, during summer break the previous year hadn't given me Potomac Fever, this second one did. It also fed into my trouble-making energy.

I was excited to be in Washington. Lyndon Johnson, a fellow Texan, was now president, and I thought for sure I should be able to get into the White House and meet him. So, one hot Washington afternoon, before I had anything else to do on that trip, 17-year-old Sam decided to go to the White House and see if President Lyndon Johnson might have a minute to meet with me. I dressed up in a suit and a tie. I walked up to a guard booth at the front of the White House, facing Pennsylvania Avenue. I said that I was there to see the President and handed the guard my John Birch Society membership card, along with my Texas driver's license. I know, yes, I too look back at that moment and wonder: "What were you thinking, Sam?"

The guard looked at my John Birch Society card, paused, and said, "Just a moment." He called someone, and as he was on the phone, I started to wonder if I might be arrested. He hung up, turned, and said that I would have to go around the corner to the visitors' entrance and sign up for a tour. I may have dodged another few hours behind bars then.

The summer-long visit with my sister, Marion, meant I needed to find something to do in Washington. Marion went to work every day, so I needed to find a job. At this point, I don't recall why we didn't get in touch with the El Paso congressman, Ed Franklin, or Senator Ralph Yarborough. Probably because we didn't know them or have any connections. Instead, I answered an ad in the newspaper. A summer job to help "give away" encyclopedias.

I was hired by a group of folks selling *Encyclopedia Britannica* door-to-door. It was, however, positioned to us as naïve young kids as "giving away" the encyclopedia, provided the household agreed to keep them updated. In high school, I would sell bags of peanuts by going door-to-door in my neighborhood in order to pay for my time at a summer camp. I did well at that! I wasn't afraid of going door-to-door to offer these encyclopedias.

When I reported to work, I found a group of young men, no women, all about my age. After about a week of training, we started "selling" and were driven to various towns in rural West Virginia. There were two men in charge, and we were split into two groups. We would go with them on the first nights, to watch them work. It would usually start around 4 or 5 p.m., or weekend nights, so folks would be at home. I'm not sure how they identified houses with children, and it might have been just looking for some external indication, like a tricycle outside or swings in the backyard. Knock on the door and say that we were here because they had been selected to receive a free encyclopedia.

It seems the folks in West Virginia were reasonable prospects for door-to-door salesmen, who claimed we were "giving away" encyclopedias. The only catch in the "gift" was the family had to agree to subscribe to a ten-year program of annual "updates," each costing a few hundred dollars. Once there was a "yes," then they told them that they would have to pay for the first three years of updates at that time. When these slick salesmen did it, they seemed to get a sale every time! It was amazing to watch. It could have been a training video; the family said *yes* to each leading question he asked. "You do want your child to do well in school, don't you?"

While my dramatic-sounding brush with the White House guard was impressive, I came to understand it as radically stupid. On the other hand, I suspect my work as a door-to-door encyclopedia "seller" influenced my eventual route to a consumer activist career.

A particular event stands out. On the initial trip of our group to West Virginia, we consisted of two adults, seven Caucasian kids, and one African American kid. Our first stop was for lunch at a downtown cafeteria in Charles Town, West Virginia. As we were all going through the cafeteria line, each of us with our cafeteria-style tray sliding along the food line, the chef/owner came out and told our manager that "he" couldn't eat there. "He" was the one African American kid with us. I had never been exposed to such blatant racism. Our manager told us to leave our trays, all 8 of them, on the counter in front of the food—exactly where they were—and leave. We all walked out, leaving those in line behind us to wait until the trays were cleared. It made a great impression on me about doing the right thing at the right time.

In retrospect, these contrasting moments in Washington, DC, between high school and college, were what I needed. My sister, Marion, was living alone at the time and once again served as an inspiring force in my life. She was the only family member that I could turn to for non-judgmental advice. Back then, Marion was breaking barriers herself. She had moved from Philadelphia, where she spent about a year with the National Student Association. Afterward, she moved to Washington, DC, and worked as a "copy girl" for the Dow Jones Company, publishers of the Wall Street Journal. In 1963, Dow Jones launched a weekly newspaper called The National Observer, and Marion secured a position as a full-time reporter there. (There is some evidence that she was the first full-time female reporter for a Dow Jones publication, other than during WWI.)

When I returned to Washington to work for Ralph Nader seven years later, 1970, Marion was still working with the *National Observer*. My work for Nader had already garnered a mention in *The New York Times*. Marion, wanting to help her brother and her paper, introduced me to one of her newspaper colleagues, who then conducted an interview with me for what turned out to be a feature article, accompanied by a picture, in *The National Observer*.

CHAPTER 6

CALMING DOWN AND FALLING IN LOVE

My own Alzheimer's journey—a counter-intuitive, counter-well-worn expectation for those with this disease—is simply an extension, I think, of my entire life. I wonder if it would have been easier if either Susan or I had experienced Alzheimer's in our families as we grew up. Neither of us did, although both of us did have someone very old in our homes. Susan's grandmother Rosie, and my grandmother Ernestine. As a result, once I was diagnosed, we were left to find our own way, figuring it out "on the go," so to speak. It now feels to me, in retrospect, that this was always a part of our entire life together. No roadmaps. Almost an improvised life—indeed, as you will discover, I did become trained in theatrical improv.

When I came home from the summer of 1963 in Washington, DC, with my sister Marion, I was ready to start college. In what turned out to be a personal style, I was determined to focus on school and get good grades—no more C- grades, my high school grade point average. It was part determination and part a lack of self-confidence. I was afraid I might not be as smart as my peers. Additionally, I wanted to earn good enough grades to secure a scholarship to the University of Texas at Austin. I was still hoping I could transfer there during either my sophomore or junior year. I would follow big sister Marion's path. I loved her independence and what seemed to me a great success. She was already working on some important stuff and getting bylines on articles in a national newspaper.

I meant business. I lived at home and studied my butt off. By the end of my first year at Texas Western, I was an A-student. It surprised me when, at first. I discovered I had one of the best academic records of any of my friends, mainly those from El Paso High, who couldn't go away to college. Academics were getting easier for me, and so I got involved in the local Jewish fraternity, Sigma Alpha Mu—ironically, we were known, in English, as Sammy's. I was still thinking about transferring to the University of Texas at Austin.

Then everything changed. I fell in love. It was during that sophomore year at Texas Western College in El Paso that I met, or re-met, Susan Meryl Kalmans. Susan was from Houston, Texas, and she ended up in El Paso, the most distant city from Houston in Texas, because she wanted to be as far away from home as possible in college. And her parents, like mine, could not afford out-of-state tuition. Well, El Paso is a 13-hour drive from Houston, damned far away. Susan's family had a cousin who lived in El Paso. Also, her oldest brother, Buddy (real name Bennet), had served a tour in the Army in El Paso. Fort Bliss is the name of the Army base in El Paso.

It turns out that I had "met" Susan before, well, sort of. Susan and I soon discovered that we had been at the same youth group convention in Texarkana, Texas, two years earlier, when we were both 16 years old. While we had noticed each other and spent some real time flirting, we never actually met. Now, we were both 18, we noticed each other again, started dating, and soon fell in love. This was now the fall of 1964, following my summer in Washington, DC.

The full story of that early romance is part of my last book, *The Actual Dance: Love's Ultimate Journey Through Breast Cancer*. The important part of that story, for the purposes of this book, is to emphasize how much our desire to get married caused me a lot of trouble.

While Susan and my relationship was starting, my trouble-making genes also began to reawaken. I got active in student government and was elected to the student senate. Then the world blew up.

It is a warm and comfortable November day in El Paso as I was heading to my freshman history class. The professor's name was Dr. Porter. Yes, it is a moment still, all these years later, as clear and real as if it were just yesterday.

I had an armful of books as I walked into the Liberal Arts Building. As I went through the front doors, I immediately sensed that something was off. A gaggle of students is darting around, many rushing toward the exits. On a typical day, they would be headed toward the classroom. I am confused and stop in my tracks. I notice a friend coming toward me. I don't remember her name. Still, 62 years later, I picture her face distorted in that moment. Hispanic, tall, slim, black hair and dark eyes, with a panicked look. Almost running, I try to stop her, and I raise my voice to ask: "What's wrong!"

She continues past as if she hadn't heard or seen me. Then she stops short, swirls around, and shouts, "The President has been shot!" Then she swirls back to run out of the building.

Unlike most other teachers in that moment, my American history professor, Dr. Porter, did not dismiss class. Instead, he delivers his prepared lecture as if everything is normal. We occasionally notice the commotion outside our classroom door. At the end of the prepared lecture, he puts down his notes. He says, "Democracies that survive best in history manage through challenging times, like the assassinations today of President Kennedy and Governor Connolly." At the time, we only knew that the governor had been shot, too. It turns out he survived.

It was, in some ways, the real beginning of the turbulent '60s. I was still tied to my dream of earning good grades, attending the University of Texas at Austin, and distancing myself from my old life in El Paso, all the while becoming more like my sister, Marion.

My folks, on the other hand, had a different vision for me. They urged me to join ROTC in college, which I did as a freshman. Like all my other courses, I worked hard to be at the top in my ROTC cohort. I excelled, or so it seems, because I applied for and received a full college scholarship from the Army. I could use it to attend any American college or university with an ROTC program. It covered both tuition and living expenses. This could have been my answer to getting out of town.

It was the first year ROTC scholarships were ever offered, and the Army was in desperate need of officers. In my parents' eyes, my future was to follow my brother-in-law, the West Point graduate, and make a career in the Army as an officer. I could retire in my 40s with a nice pension and do whatever I wanted after that.

I had two different models in front of me: my oldest sister, Marion, who, after going to the University of Texas at Austin, was able to go to work for the then thought to be radical-left advocacy group, The National Student Association (NSA). I don't think I mentioned that she went to Europe for a time, while at NSA, and I would later—like 40 years later—learn that she had become pregnant and had a baby that was put up for adoption. It was pretty troublemaking stuff in the 1950s and early '60s.

The other model was Evelyn, two years younger than Marion, and a contrast to her older sister. Evelyn did not finish college, married a West Point cadet at 18, and was pregnant by the time she was 19. As my college days progressed, my parents pushed me hard to take the Evelyn path. I was buying in a bit. Mainly because I was falling in love with Susan, and as time moved on, we both, Susan and I, were also caught up in illnesses in both families—Susan's mother was very sick with breast cancer by then, and my dad had suffered his stroke and was out of work for a bit.

Which model would I follow? My trouble-making urges were being stoked in different ways during this time. During the 1960s, the opposition to the Vietnam War and the politicians who supported it was fierce. The battle for racial justice was in full swing—the MLK March on Washington and the Vietnam War dominated the news. My sister Harriet visited my sister in Marion in Washington, and they were both at the Washington Mall for the MLK March and his famous speech. My best friend, Ken, was a "Peacenik" and very active in the local Texas Western campus anti-war movement. In retrospect, I love the incongruity of having been a leader in ROTC and having a best friend who was a leader in the anti-war student movement. It was a profoundly important lifelong lesson to me that such a thing was, in fact, possible. Ken eventually left the country to live in Canada. We still see each other as best friends.

By the time we were second-semester sophomore students, at the start of 1964, Susan and I were a couple. Love decided how I would live the rest of my life. No, even with the ROTC scholarship, I would not leave El Paso. I needed to be with Susan.

We both wanted to get married. We had already gone from dating to going steady. Then I gave Susan my fraternity ring to wear on a necklace. In college, that ring around the neck, often referred to as "pre-engaged," signaled an intent to propose marriage.

As it turns out, we split the difference between Marion and Evelyn. Like Evelyn and her husband Gene, Susan and I end up marrying very young. Like Marion, I end up causing trouble. Indeed, even our decision to get married ended up causing trouble.

CHAPTER 7

A GREAT PLAN UNTIL IT WASN'T

Our future seemed all set. Susan and Sam—in love as sophomores in college. I was an A student and had just received the ROTC scholarship. Despite our parents' efforts to slow us down, we had "hooked up"—also known as having sex—and we wanted to get married. Our future seemed ordinary and clear. Yet the seeds of a different path had already been planted, and a different future was lurking in the background.

I remember my mother pleading, almost begging, with me to break up with Susan. "Wait a while, Sam. Meet other girls! If it is true love, you two will get back together." I argued, and I persisted. My persistent argumentation was not the real reason my parents finally relented and agreed to our marriage in 1966, while Susan was still 20 and I was 21. The real reason was something more urgent and compelling.

Susan's mother's breast cancer had spread throughout her body. Her doctors did not know how long she would survive, and Susan and her family wanted her mother to be able to walk down the aisle as her youngest child was getting married. Considering this development, my parents said that we could get married on one condition: we would have to be able to support ourselves. We accepted the challenge and developed a plan. Susan would attend summer school and complete her credits during the summer of her third year of college. We would then get married. She had secured a job as a kindergarten teacher in the El Paso public school system, starting in the fall. I would continue in school and get a part-time job selling men's clothing at Al's Shop for Men. Al, being Al Weiss, a member of our reform temple, also hired a few other young men from Temple Mount Sinai to work part-time. I spoke to him, and he assured me of a continued opportunity and that he would give me priority to work the hours I needed.

Yes, we could do it! Yes, we did. On August 23, 1966, we were married in Houston, Texas, at Beth Yeshurun synagogue in the Greenfield Chapel. Susan's mother walked down the aisle. She got to see her youngest daughter get married.

We were starry-eyed kids, excited and looking forward to a life together. Despite the wedding and our joy of the moment, we sensed that no one thought it was a good idea or that our marriage would last. As I mentioned, Susan and I just hit the 59th-year mark of our marriage. At some point, the number becomes irrelevant; it is as if it has always been this way.

We started that first year of marriage. Susan worked for the public schools, and I was in college, working part-time at Al's Shop for Men, and in an elite ROTC group with a vision for perhaps a career in the Army. I had received that full ROTC academic scholarship starting in my junior year of college on the condition that I would first be able to go to law school. So, yes, a career in the Army would still be possible as a lawyer. In the Army, it is called the Judge Advocate General's Corps. In the meantime, I would avoid being a second lieutenant infantryman in Vietnam at the height of the war.

We had a plan: I would obtain a deferment to attend law school and then fulfill my military obligation as a lawyer. Then have an option to stay or leave. I applied to the University of Texas School of Law (UT Law) in Austin and got accepted. My start date would be September 1967.

While all this was happening, the opposition to the Vietnam War and the military continued to explode on campuses throughout the United States. I was living within a complex web of life connections and loyalties. On one end were my parents and their visions for me, and the model of my sister and her West Point husband already in the Army. On the other hand, there was my best friend, Ken, a leader in the local anti-war movement, and the news filled with dying soldiers and stories of growing anti-war sentiment. My sympathies lay with Ken. I believed that the Vietnam War was wrong.

Two incidents during this time impacted my future life choices.

First, Ken was part of the activist anti-war group, and one day, he and others demonstrated against the war in downtown El Paso at Plaza Park. It was the center of downtown EL Paso, where most city bus lines terminated. I had taken the Mesita bus to attend the City Council meeting to protest the 11 p.m. curfew back in 1957. Now, in the 1960s, this was where Ken Goldberg and other anti-war advocates went to protest the Vietnam War.

The protestors walked in a large circle around the perimeter of the park with anti-war signs. A crowd began to gather, mainly folks who supported the war. I was, of course, there again to support Ken. Some people started calling the students traitors, and others began to jump in as they passed by and threw punches at the demonstrators, who eventually had to flee for safety.

Not long after, on campus at Texas Western, Ken and his anti-war friends decided to hold an educational event on the patio of the school's Student Union building. They put up three long portable tables with literature. The idea was to provide people with anti-war materials, essentially a brochure, and discuss the war with them. Again, I show up to support Ken, who was one of several activists standing behind the tables, ready to hand out the brochure and have a conversation.

Sensing a mob forming behind me, I decide to step up to the table, and pick up the literature as an example, at least in my mind, of what to do. How to behave. I call it a mob because I could feel the heat of their hate. Without even looking, I can sense danger. I am alone at the table, looking at the material, when suddenly an arm shoves past my waist, under the table in front of me, and flips it over on its side.

Literature flies all over the place. The demonstrators flee for safety into the student Union building. I flee with them.

Our school president rushed to the scene, stands atop the rock wall, and gives an impromptu lecture on free speech. The event makes national news, and a picture of the school president appears in Newsweek! An indelible moment for me. Interestingly, I wasn't one of the troublemakers at the time, although I was standing with them. Indeed, I'm almost the one who got run over by the crowd that day, and I ran away with the troublemakers.

At this point in my journey, I was more concerned about the war and the possibility now that I might end up in combat in Vietnam and be killed than I was about emulating my West Point brother-in-law. I was still that 90-pound weakling. Okay, I was 6'2" and I weighed 130 pounds. I smoked. I was not athletic in any way. Yes, I could march in my ROTC uniform and carry an old rifle. I could not do any sit-ups, nor run any distance.

"Go to law school," I remember as a "what else am I going to do" thought. It was also a path into the political world and advocacy, a growing interest of mine. I could still go to the Army. I made sure when I accepted the ROTC scholarship that I would still be eligible to get a deferment for graduate school, if I wanted it. And now I did.

I did. I applied to the University of Texas School of Law, where almost every in-state applicant was accepted. Although my grade point average was A-, I was not accepted on the first round. I think I didn't do well on the LSAT test. I got the acceptance letter by the winter of my senior year.

Unfortunately, by then, the US Army changed its mind about deferments.

The war in Vietnam wasn't going well, and the Army needed more second Lieutenants. Too many were being killed at the time, often by their own men who thought them incompetent. The Army decided to revoke my deferment and required me to proceed directly to active duty. I was assigned to the infantry, and my initial post would be to attend the Army Infantry School in Fort Benning, Georgia.

I objected and decided to cause some trouble. I had an ally in that troublemaking. My ROTC professor (or PMS—professor of military science) remembered our conversation when I asked if the scholarship would affect my ability to attend graduate school. He had assured me it would not. Now he was mortified about the change in policy and offered to facilitate an appeal of the decision to revoke my deferment.

It was the summer of 1967, and Susan and I had, upon graduation, moved from El Paso to an apartment in Houston to be near her mother. Her mother's breast cancer was advancing, and the end was near. At the same time, we were awaiting the decision on what was next in our lives: law school or Ft. Benning, Georgia.

On August 5th, the phone rang in our apartment. Her brother was calling to tell her: "It is time." Susan needed to get to the hospital and join her father, two brothers, and her oldest sister. Her mother was ready to take her last breath. I sat in the hospital waiting room as Susan, her sister Bernice, and two brothers, Melvin and Buddy, went into the hospital room. About half an hour later, they came out together. I hugged Susan, and we all went to our respective homes.

On the funeral day, two days later, the family had gathered after the burial at Susan's growing-up home for the mourners' meal. It was a busy room, I didn't know all the people, and was a bit off to the side, when someone came up to me and said there was a long-distance phone call for me. It was my mother calling.

I had not been aware of my father's recent hospitalization, and Mom was in tears. "You need to come home, Sam, right away. Your father is not expected to survive." I started to object. I was comforting Susan, and I was confused about what to do. In a harsh voice, my mother barked, "Sam, *your family* needs you."

I rushed to El Paso, and on August 14th, nine days after Susan's mother's death, my father, Marcus, passed away. Susan flew into El Paso for the funeral. We still had not heard from the Army. We returned to Houston to mark our first wedding anniversary on August 23, 1967. Susan's grandmother, Grandma Rosie Kalmans, gave us some money to go out to dinner, and then made sure we were able to go back to Susan's home to enjoy the unfrozen top layer of what had been our wedding cake. I'm not sure if this is still a custom—freeze the top layer of the wedding cake to be eaten on the first wedding anniversary. ChatGPT tells me it still is.

Yes, on August 23, 1967, we still waited to find out what was next in our lives. Where would we be in three weeks? My hope: Law school in Austin, Texas, at the University of Texas. Or would it be Fort Benning, Georgia, Infantry School, and then me off to Vietnam? In my view, a death sentence.

Then late one morning, about one week later, the telephone rang. "Lt. Simon, this is the office of the Vice-Chief of Staff of the US Army, calling to let you know that as an exception to standing policy, your deferment to attend law school has been granted."

A life-altering—if not lifesaving—phone call.

CHAPTER 8

STARTING A CAREER AS A TROUBLEMAKER

I entered law school at the University of Texas in Austin in the fall of 1967 with the same energy I had entered undergraduate school in El Paso four years earlier. I was determined to get good grades. I was also terrified that I would not be able to compete with the numerous Harvard and Yale graduates in our class. The result was I did *nothing* other than study for my entire first year of law school. Once again, Susan made it all possible. She worked, and we were able to secure a loan that would not have to be repaid until after law school.

When I say I did nothing but study, I mean I was obsessed. Law students and lawyers will understand the level because they understand what it takes to outline every case in our casebooks. No one ever did that, I was told. Yet, I did!

Was that obsession and determination to do well, to beat the odds, a reflection of the energy that would also develop around fighting for justice, causing trouble in my career and life? Never satisfied, nor secure, always seeking the best or maybe the fairest outcomes possible.

The obsession to outline every case in the textbook did help. I also learned something else that surprised me. I had a natural aptitude for the law—I "thought like a lawyer." I found that students with highly structured thought processes or who were really good in math and sciences tended to struggle in law school. A lot of those top Ivy League undergraduate students did poorly, ending up in the middle of our class. Those of us with more liberal arts backgrounds, who could see all sides of an issue or a problem, tended to do better.

I surprised myself. All three years of law school, I ended up at the very top of my class. At the University of Texas School of Law, the typical grade for a course was "C." I was not only usually a "B," I even earned an "A" in Constitutional Law class. Almost unheard of! I was eligible for the Law Review—students who edited and published a quarterly book of legal articles by both students and professors. I graduated in the top 10th percentile, with honors in a class that had more than 400 students in its first year. I was also awarded membership in "The Order of The Coif," the highest honorary distinction for a graduating law school student. Yes, I thought like a lawyer.

Three events during this time presaged what would become my life as a troublemaker in Washington, DC.

The first was another chance to spend the summer in Washington, DC, reminiscent of my summer seven years earlier, after graduating from high school. Except now I was 23 years old and married. I secured an internship for the summer of 1969 at the Office of the General Counsel of the Department of the Navy. My oldest sister, Marion, still lived in DC, and was now married. Susan and I spent this summer living in the basement of her townhouse on Monroe Street in the inner city of Washington, DC.

This is near where the riots of 1968 occurred following the assassination of Martin Luther King. My sister assured us that the then mainly African American neighborhood was safe. I was working in the center of DC in an old World War II office building on the Washington Mall. Susan got a summer job working as a cashier at a Cadillac car dealership.

We were exposed to a city and a time when racial unrest still sat just below the surface. I can still recall the energy I felt about wanting to be part of the solution, even though my work was unrelated to any of that. I think this might be when I caught the Washington bug, the knowing I would need to come back to this place.

We returned to Austin for my third and final year of law school. There was, and probably still is, a saying that in law school, the first year, they scare you to death, and yes, I outlined every case. The second year, they work you to death, and yes, I worked my butt off when I was back for that second year. It didn't leave me that much time for troublemaking. In the third year, supposedly, they bore you to death.

Well, not me, because during my third year, I was causing trouble again. My grades made me eligible for the Law Review. I wrote an article for the Review, a requirement for those of us selected to be members, in which I advocated for laws to allow tenants in rental properties to unionize: Tenant Unions. It turns out that this concept was similar to an idea that Ralph Nader—my future boss—was developing. He called them CUBS. Those initials referred to Citizen Utility Boards. These would be non-profit advocacy organizations made up of customers of various companies, mainly utility customers. Customers would be allowed to choose to add a small payment to their utility bill to fund a Consumer Office. The group would then represent ratepayer interests at the State utility commissions.

Ralph Nader had a variation of the idea for all sorts of consumer-funded organizations with a mandate to represent the consumer's interests in regulatory proceedings. The big idea was to create a student organization on a college campus to advocate for and support student-proposed issues and positions, as determined by the students. Even in the TV industry, Ralph advocated for viewers and listeners to form "The Audience Network." Viewers would be allowed to create an Audience Network organization that would own a broadcast period during prime time. Ralph wanted an hour a night for their programming to reach and organize viewers to be advocates in Washington. Like Public Broadcasting, they could also raise money for their work by asking for support on the TV programs they would produce.

My idea, which I had before working for Ralph, was to allow tenants to organize themselves like unions to negotiate with the landlord, and to advocate for tenant rights. Ralph loved that idea, too. Years later, meaning now, I'm joining all sorts of emerging organizations made up of people with dementia or Alzheimer's Disease that let us raise our voices directly. It used to be that there was only the Alzheimer's Association, which has grown very large, and to some, is more corporate than grassroots. There was big Pharma—the maker of drugs who often pretended to speak in "our voice'—those with disease.

The newer patient groups are smaller and often led or governed by individuals with cognitive disorders, or their caregivers.

In my third year of law school, "bored to death" as the saying went, I spent my time with other troublemakers in our class. We had formed a bond. A small group in the class of 1970 was aligned with advocacy and more progressive causes. As it turns out, anti-Vietnam War protests that had been starting back when I was in college were now erupting across the United States, especially on university campuses. At Kent State University in Ohio, four students were killed by the police, and nine others were wounded in the shooting. In Austin that same year, a large protest was planned, and the Austin City Council refused to grant a parade permit. They instead called out the State Police. Everyone was sure there would be a repeat of Kent State and possible violence. Tens of thousands of people were coming to Austin. Without the parade permit, they would have to stay on the sidewalks.

It seemed obvious that there would be a serious clash with the police, that violence could erupt, and that people could be killed. At the time, I and several members of the

Texas Law Review and a professor decided to do something to force the city to issue the parade permit. We stayed up all night to file a *Writ of Mandamus*, asking a court to order the city to issue the parade permit in accordance with the 1st Amendment. We won, and a *writ of mandamus* was issued right before the march itself was about to start. Crowds of people were gathering on the sidewalks, while fully geared State Police were feet away just waiting for people to get into the streets.

That morning, as I walked home, not having slept, I watched as the crowd got the news of the court decision forcing the permit to be granted, and left sidewalks, spreading out into the street. It had a profound emotional impact on me and the power of the law for a just cause.

There was one other crucial troublemaking project. My constitutional law professor recommended me to a local Austin lawyer who was working pro bono (free) on a case to have the Texas poll tax declared unconstitutional. It happens that my "final" paper in that constitutional law class was an argument on why the poll tax was unconstitutional. He had given me an "A"! Again, one of those grades is almost never awarded to a student.

A bit of background for this generation. At one time, many states, primarily Southern states, imposed a "fee" that voters had to pay to participate in an election. Texas had such a fee. The lawyer represented a group of low-income individuals who sought to have the law declared unconstitutional and required assistance with researching and drafting the brief. I did research and early drafting, and the case was won. Eventually, the Supreme Court of the United States upheld similar cases and outlawed poll taxes nationwide.

As graduation from law school was nearing, I was again at a turning point. What should I do? What were my choices? A phrase that oddly reappeared shortly after I was diagnosed with Alzheimer's disease. The stakes are, in fact, almost identical. Life or death. As you have read, shortly after getting my diagnosis, I discovered the movement advocating for assisted suicide for those with Alzheimer's and similar disorders. There was and is an argument being made that life with this disease is not worth living. Legislation is being proposed and passed in a number of states that allows for assisted suicide for those who want to die earlier and earlier in the process.

The choices—the "what are my choices"—issue was not at that moment considered life and death, though they were about the meaning and purpose of life. Graduating from UT Law in the late 1960s into the '70s, there was a new language about choices for graduates. Especially for those of us from the Law Review with excellent resumes and lots of choices. We could take "the golden train" from Austin (Law School) to Houston.

Houston, the largest city in the state, was also the home of the largest and most prestigious law firms in Texas. Even though I had my Army obligation, I applied to a couple of the big law firms and was invited to an interview at one of the largest firms. I was interviewed by several lawyers, then treated to an elaborate private lunch with several of the firm's senior partners. I was different because if they wanted me, they would need to wait until after my military tour. I did not get a job offer from them.

A series of events unfolded, however, that set my destiny. First, shortly before I visited Houston for the elaborate big-law firm interview, the *Texas Law Review* hosted its annual dinner with a featured speaker—a Texas law graduate named Nicholas (Nick) Johnson. Nick had graduated from UT Law and immediately went to Washington, DC, to become a troublemaker extraordinaire. He was the youngest person ever to serve as the administrator of the US Maritime Commission. President Lyndon Johnson appointed him, and then, when Nick ended up causing that industry so much trouble, the President "transferred him," in effect, by appointing him to the Federal Communications Commission. No, the two Johnsons were not related.

I don't know the story of how Nicholas, who was from Iowa, was able to snag these appointments. In thinking back to these times, it is almost eerie—as if foreshadowing the inevitability of my career. Nick became a member of the Federal Communications Commission in 1966 and served until 1973. In 1970, he published a book called *How to Talk Back to Your Television Set* (Little Brown, January 1970). He was the one who urged us law review students not to take the Golden Train and instead to work in the public interest world. Nick eventually played an even more significant role in my troublemaker life.

About a decade later, I would become the executive director of a consumer group that had been led for a time by the same Nick Johnson. It turns out that Nick Johnson and Ralph Nader had become buddies in Washington, DC. Around 1979, Nick lost interest in the group. It was a time when several public interest groups were going under, and Ralph offered to take it over if I would agree to lead it and if Nick would at least stay on as a member of the board of directors.

Of course, that was all going to be in the future. In this moment, back in my last year of law school, I was sitting in the room being inspired by the voice of Nicholas Johnson to work in the public interest, not for big law firms. Of course, I was looking first at four years in the Army Judge Advocate General Corps. Nick, though, stoked the troublemaker spark that was brewing inside.

As I said, that point in law school, I was part of a small group of politically liberal or progressive students. My closest friends in school were, like me, politically progressive. There were three in particular: Jim Welch, Peter Petkas, and Joe Tom Easley. Peter and Jim were classmates, and Joe Tom, while older, was a year behind us.

It turns out that in the summer of 1969, when I was in Washington, DC, interning at the Department of the Navy, Joe Tom was also in Washington working for the emerging celebrity Ralph Nader. Nader had hired law students every summer since 1967 to descend into Washington, DC, and investigate federal agencies. They had become known as "Nader's Raiders." Joe Tom was a "Raider" that summer of 1969. He returned to school to tell us that Ralph Nader was planning to start a new public-interest law firm called The Public Interest Research Group (PIRG). He encouraged

Jim, Peter, and me to apply and recommended us to Ralph. Ralph and Joe Tom had bonded during that summer, and Ralph trusted Joe Tom. Indeed, eventually, Joe Tom narrated an HBO-aired film about Ralph's life called *An Unreasonable Man*.

Of course, troublemaker Sam was interested in working for Ralph Nader. The question was how I could manage my Army obligation and take a job working with Ralph Nader in Washington, DC. Plus, Susan and I had already become pregnant with our son. We'd planned for the baby to be born while I was in the Army, thus having them pay the medical costs.

It turns out that the obligation for the Nader job at PIRG required only a one-year commitment. I did not know then that Ralph planned to use this initial group as a test bed for public interest advocacy in Washington, DC, and beyond. The opportunity enticed me, and my law school success and activities ended my vision of a career in the Army.

I decided to apply. First, though, I called folks within the US Army and asked if my active-duty reporting date could be deferred until 1971. "Not a problem," they said, if I could report by April 1971. I had a plan. Graduate and report to work for Ralph on July 1, 1970, and be part of the very first Public Interest Research Group until April 1971. It would work out, but not exactly that way.

My job interview with Nader was conducted over the telephone. As I understood it, Ralph was at a payphone in the hallway of his apartment building. He must have been well-briefed, because he immediately offered me the job. The fact that I had to enter the Army in April and could not stay until July 1971 didn't bother him. He would pay me the full $2,400, 12-month stipend anyway. I was delighted and felt like a hotshot. After all, I had just learned that I was graduating in the top 10 percent of my class. While that might have helped, I suspect it was the recommendation from Joe Tom Easley, my classmate, that made the difference. I have also learned that several of my colleagues in that year had the same experience. A quick interview and a quick offer. At least I knew, and at the end of the conversation, that I had been offered a job. Some of the others who were hired said they had not realized that Ralph had offered them the job on the spot, so to speak, until weeks later!

For me, Sam Simon, that moment, that decision, set the path for the rest of my professional life, if not everything else about my life. It also resulted in a lifetime relationship between Ralph Nader and me, and both of our families. Even today, as I write this, Ralph and I have "business" together.

My reckless nature was setting off alarm bells within the family. Susan's parents were beside themselves with anxiety. I was taking a job with this crazy, in-the-headlines, controversial guy while their daughter was pregnant. I didn't have any idea how I was going to pay for the birth. Plus, I would now be in Washington, DC, taking the bar exam on the day the baby was due. Also, the lease on the apartment we lived in was going to run out, so we took a motel room to live in temporarily. Susan's oldest sister, Bernice, came to Austin, Texas, from Brownsville, where she lived, to be with Susan while she gave birth. Or so we thought.

As it turned out, our son-to-be didn't want to be born on the planned date. Indeed, the first attempt at birth showed that he had not fully turned in the womb, and Susan would need a Caesarean Section. I was able to get back to Austin in time for the C-section and the birth of our now 55-year-old son, Marcus. And yes, our son is also a bit of a troublemaker. An elected member of the Virginia House of Delegates representing the Falls Church, Virginia area. As I write this, he is 26th in seniority of a 100-member chamber.

Of course, the story does not end without my causing the hospital a little trouble. I showed up to check Susan and our new son out of the hospital. There was a window with a sign "Pay Here." There was no line, so I walked up, gave my name, and they handed me the bill. We didn't have enough money to pay it. Yes, even at 25, with a law degree, I asked if they would let Susan and our new son, Marcus, leave the hospital if I couldn't pay the bill! Yes, I could. They were not going to be held as collateral!

The next nine months in Washington, DC, were a deep initiation into big-time troublemaking. Working as part of a "first" in Washington, DC, at the start of the 1970s in a high-visibility project. Nader himself was still an emerging national phenomenon. All it took for us—about 15 new lawyers—to get through to whomever we wanted in Washington, DC, was to say that we were calling from Ralph Nader's office. "This is Sam Simon, calling from Ralph Nader's office. Is Senator Johnson available?" The answer was almost always, Yes!

It was the job of a lifetime. I believe that even today, 55 years later. The work we did got us a lot of attention. Not long after I reported for work, there was a moment, not unlike that all-nighter in law school the previous year, when we sued the city of Austin to get the parade permit. Except this time, we were going to sue the president of the United States. Once again, one of the other lawyers and I stayed up all night drafting a lawsuit, this time against President Richard Nixon.

Yes, again, we won! At least temporarily, we halted the implementation of a regulation granting massive tax breaks to large businesses because President Nixon had not complied with the Administrative Procedures Act, which mandated a public rulemaking process to change the rules. The court invalidated the Executive Order and required the President to run his proposed new regulations through the Administrative Procedures Act process. The court agreed that the president wasn't a dictator and had to follow the law.

Suing the President was much more fun than what turned out to be my main project for Ralph. It was just an unexpectedly exciting opportunity. How often does a lawyer get to sue the President of the United States and win? I believe these early experiences have helped me throughout my life to have the courage to challenge norms and exceed expectations. It is particularly helpful now with my Alzheimer's. Who could imagine that choosing to write and perform a play would be possible after being diagnosed with Alzheimer's?

My principal project for Nader in 1970 was more mundane. I oversaw the "Property Tax Project." Our goal was to end the practices of giant corporations abusing their economic power to extort taxing authorities into granting large property tax breaks. It was a common practice at the time, and still is, to some extent, for the largest corporations. Our goal was to draw national attention to the practice and urge States to enact legislation to limit corporate power.

My project got a lot of attention. The Property Tax Conference was held in the fall of 1970, and our keynote speaker was then US Senator Ed Muskie. At the time, Muskie was considered a potential Presidential candidate for the 1972 ticket. We got some attention!

Indeed, my work got me featured in an article in the *New York Times* business section written by Eileen Shannahan, who later became the *Times'* Washington bureau chief. Eileen happened to meet my wife and our newborn son, during that interview. She was taken by our story and referred us to a *New York Times'* Style Section reporter, Nan Robertson. Nan visited us in our one-bedroom apartment, with no television, and wrote a profile piece headlined, "Nader Raiding is No Plush Job" in 1971. It appeared on the front page of the Style section of the *Times* with a picture of me, Susan, and baby Marcus. We were getting known nationwide as a troublemaking family.

The pattern of working for the public interest, challenging norms—let's say causing trouble—was well set. Or let's say, just beginning on a grander scale. I was the first person in that 1970 group to leave Ralph because I had that military commitment. In April of 1971, I entered the U.S. Army as a Captain in the Judge Advocate General's Corps. My assignment was in the Judge Advocate's office at Fort Lee, Virginia, located just outside Petersburg, Virginia, approximately a two-hour drive from Washington, DC. Fort Lee was renamed Fort Gregg-Adams in 2021 in honor of two African American officers. Lt. General Arthur J. Gregg (second lieutenant at the time) had been denied access to the officers' club in 1950 at a time when discrimination and segregation were still widespread. Lt. Colonel Charity Adams (1918–2002) fought against segregation in the Army. She is portrayed in a 2024 film. The original name was in honor of Robert E. Lee, the head of the Confederacy. The Fort Lee name was restored in 2025, following the re-election of Donald Trump.

Remembering we had wanted the Army to pay for the birth of our children, Susan and I got busy trying to make another baby. Our daughter, Rachael Laura Simon, now 54 as I write this, was born there, at the then Ft. Lee, Virginia hospital. It was also there that we learned Susan had significant uterine fibroids, and with her mother's history of cancer, we made the decision to have her uterus removed. We had a boy and a girl; that had been our plan from the beginning.

It was not quite a year into my service at Fort Lee when the Army began to feel the edges of my elbows—aka "troublemaking." In retrospect, it was inevitable I would cause the Army (and myself) trouble, given my life history up to that time and my high-visibility role as a Ralph Nader consumer advocate.

A little background. The Judge Advocate General's Corps supports the legal needs of the US Army across the world. In the United States, that involves the equivalent of a local "law office" or a city attorney's office. Among the various duties for the lawyers would be to provide legal advice to the base commander. Similarly, legal advice to other "businesses" or operations on the base that do things like contract for supplies, landlord-tenant issues around base housing, and so forth.

My initial work was to review contracts and advise on procurement issues. It was not so fraught and not so time-consuming. Perhaps that is why I was assigned to represent an Army officer in an administrative matter. It was my first trial-like case as a lawyer. I represented an Army captain being discharged from the Army for cause—"failure to keep pace with contemporaries." It turns out that when he had been in combat in Vietnam, he was courageous. Indeed, he had received various medals for bravery. However, when not in combat, he was just a pain in the ass.

In other words, he, too, was a troublemaker, of sorts, with strong opinions about everything and wasn't shy about sharing them. (Sound familiar?) He would complain to anyone about what he saw as a problem, from lack of readiness in his unit to how the barracks weren't clean enough. For example, he once berated a general, the commander of the base where he was stationed, at a public social event, for what he deemed to be the poor maintenance of the base's tanks.

His lawyer, me, wasn't shy either. We were perhaps the perfect match for this case. I suspect a more seasoned JAG officer or one who was not themselves a troublemaker could have persuaded him not to fight the discharge. It is a simple argument: "Don't appeal this because even if you 'win', you will never be promoted again." Troublemaker Sam was empathetic about his outrage. I jumped in with both feet. In fact, I represented him so well that the Army dropped its case. Ultimately, as predicted, he retired from the Army years later, still as a captain. He was never again promoted.

The next big troublemaking event for Captain Simon was something that so upset the US Army, they wanted to court-martial me. Yes, me! Talk about real trouble. In the mid-'70s the Army had a drug problem with their enlisted folks, so the President, Nixon again, declared a drug amnesty program and encouraged soldiers using drugs to turn themselves in to get help, and not be court-martialed.

My client, a young African American soldier, came to our office for help because he was about to be administratively discharged from the Army under less-than-honorable conditions. He knew that his failure to receive an honorable discharge would be a permanent stain on his reputation and impact him for the rest of his life.

The young man told me that he had been lured to turn himself in because he would occasionally use some marijuana, and he didn't want to be court-martialed. True to their word, the Army did not court-martial him. Instead, they started a procedure to administratively discharge him from the Army, citing the drug use, and insisting that he be discharged under less-than-honorable conditions. Not having an honorable discharge typically prevents someone from securing a decent job in civilian life. He knew that.

I sought to represent him. I was told to drop the matter because the discharge was "administrative," and he wasn't entitled to an Army lawyer. I protested inside the Army and got nowhere. I was outraged. So, troublemaker Sam drafted an article about what was happening to these young soldiers and submitted it to *The Nation* magazine. I also submitted it, at the same time, to the Army for their approval. I got a yes from *The Nation* magazine, but I hadn't heard from the Army yet. I did not want to lose the opportunity with *The Nation*. I approved their proposed edits, and just hoped the Army would be okay. In any case, I thought this was sort of like the Pentagon Papers, and I had a First Amendment right to speak. The Army hadn't even gotten back to me at the time the article appeared in the magazine. Boy, was I, once again, in trouble.

The Army wanted to court-martial me. I first heard about that from my boss at the time, a major. Then, someone from the Army's office of the Judge Advocate General called and asked me if my article had been intended to be a "letter to the editor." It turns out that there was an exception to "prior approval" for Letters to the Editor. So, for the first, and so far, the only time in my life, I had to invoke the 5th Amendment. "I am afraid I can't answer that question, Sir." Talk about being in some real trouble.

A happy ending of sorts. I received an official written reprimand from a general in the Army, and that reprimand was placed in my official personnel file, accompanied by an unofficial *"attaboy"* footnote. My boss, the major, called me into his office, showed me the letter of reprimand, then declared the meeting over, and told me, "The judge advocate general has asked me to tell you, 'Good job.' He wants you to know that he thinks the Army needs more advocates like you." He then pointedly said that was "off the record."

The next thing that happened was the Army got me out of the field and back to Washington, DC, to work in the Office of the Chief Trial Attorney, which was in Northern Virginia, near where we used to live. It was rumored that a friend of Ralph Nader, someone on Capitol Hill, whom Ralph had mentioned my troubles to, made some calls to a senior Pentagon official on my behalf.

Troublemaking paid off! I got a prestigious position that lets me cause even more trouble, except now *for* the Army. I was now representing the US Army, defending them against lawsuits brought by many of the largest government contractors who were suing the Army. I won some big cases.

As I write this memoir, however, events of our day—now more than fifty years later—evoke in me a sense of not having done enough for some of my clients. Especially that young man who received a discharge "under less-than-honorable conditions."

The issue of wrongful administrative discharges under less-than-honorable conditions is now back in the news. The military during the Clinton years adopted a policy to deal with the fact that, at one time, gay individuals were not allowed to serve in the military. President Clinton adopted a policy of "Don't Ask and Don't Tell". Gender status wasn't going to be a matter of discussion. Soldiers didn't need to say if they were gay. Still, there were people in the military who did tell or were "discovered" and were administratively discharged under less-than-honorable conditions. The Pentagon is now reviewing the records of those individuals and updating their status to "honorable."

I don't know whether, currently, with my Alzheimer's, I have the energy or capacity to take on that issue. I would like to see it fixed. I hope maybe I can find a politician, or just someone in the Pentagon, to start reviewing the cases from back then and change the discharges to honorable.

When I left the Army in 1974—with an honorable discharge—I once again made a modest attempt at a normal life. I wanted some security for two children, one 3 years old and one 4 years old. Susan was a stay-at-home mother, and we needed good family insurance and benefits. With two years of experience in the Army spent at the top tier of government contract litigation, I was lured to work for a prestigious law firm in Washington, DC—Fried, Frank, Harris, Shriver and Kampelman. Let's see, that's Patricia Harris, the first African American Secretary of Health and Human Services, Sargent Shriver, brother-in-law to President Kennedy, among other things, and Max Kampelman, who became US Ambassador to Russia. Not bad company.

During all this time, I kept in touch with Ralph Nader and my colleagues from that first-year PIRG experience. Ralph kept messing with my life and career. So, while I was a lawyer in a highly prestigious Washington law firm, Ralph recommended me to a brand-new US senator, John Durkin, from New Hampshire. John Durkin was also a troublemaker. I was hired as his legislative director, the second most senior position in the office. Then, when President Jimmy Carter was elected, I was recruited to work for the Federal Trade Commission as a GS-15. It was, both in that day and for me, "real money," like $78,000 a year; plus, if I stayed 20 years, there would be a federal pension. Once again, I was pulled to that place as if by a magnet to the iron of my parents' vision for my life.

Susan wasn't by nature a stay-at-home mom. Nope, as soon as our two children were eligible for daycare, she was back teaching. So, our two-salary family was doing better financially than ever. In the late '70s, our combined salary was nearly $100,000. At that moment, we were comfortably upper-class. In today's dollars, according to most calculators, that would be the equivalent to an annual income of over $600,000. I recall thinking while in law school that I would be happy if I could earn just $15,000 a year.

Naturally, we took a big step and bought a home in McLean, Virginia. The highest-scale zip code in the Virginia suburban area of DC. Yes, we were living both of our parents' dreams for a safe and secure home and family. A government job, where I could retire with a fat government pension. Susan as a teacher, who would also be able to (and did) retire with a pension. We had a beautiful home. We were members of a Reform Jewish synagogue—one where we both would become leaders. Oh, the house we bought was two doors from that of my older sister Evelyn, whose husband was a

West Point graduate and, by then, a lieutenant colonel. (He would eventually retire as a major general.) Family, security, and community, and we were still in our 30s!

Then Nicholas Johnson reappeared in my life, and it was a key factor in changing everything. Yes, that "Don't take the Golden Train to Houston," Nicolas Johnson, who was the guest speaker at the Law Review dinner in Austin in 1970. It didn't take long. It was about 1978, and we were enjoying our new house, and I had a great job. Of course, the embers of my troublemaker genes never went out. Though they may have cooled for a while; they were still burning.

It is late one evening, and I am at home, probably getting ready for bed. Ralph Nader had a reputation of calling people at any time, day or night. As was his style, Ralph calls me around 11 p.m. out of the blue. We hadn't talked in a while. He tells me that a consumer group involved in communications issues, mainly broadcast issues, was about to collapse. He wants me to leave the Federal Trade Commission and become executive director of the collapsing organization.

As an enticement, Ralph said he would serve as board chairman of the organization if I said yes. It turns out that Nicholas Johnson, yes, that Nick Johnson, had been serving as the executive director and wanted to leave the organization. As a further enticement to me, Ralph said that if I took the position, not only would he be chair of the board, Nick would also stay on as a board member and help with fundraising.

The organization we are talking about was known as the National Citizens Committee for Broadcasting (NCCB).

NCCB's original purpose was to advocate for Congress to create the Corporation for Public Broadcasting (CPB). Yes, the one that, while I'm writing this book, Congress has defunded. NCCB was a non-profit with an official committee, important people who let NCCB use their name in support of Public Broadcasting and the creation of the Corporation for Public Broadcasting. Members of the committee included some very high-profile folks like Walter Cronkite, the iconic CBS news anchor, Benjamin Hooks, the long-time head of the NAACP, Thomas Hoving, Chairman of the NY Met and son of the founder of Tiffany's, and the former Chairman of the FCC, Newton Minnow, among many other noted academics and other non-profit leaders.

NCCB was successful in its campaign. Congress created the Corporation for Public Broadcasting, which then developed the modern American public media infrastructure. Having accomplished its original mission, the NCCB underwent a transition. Rather than disbanding entirely, with support from the Benton family, now the Benton Foundation, it continued. Our friend, Nick Johnson, left the Federal Communications Commission to head the "new" NCCB, which would become the grassroots organizing arm of a new and growing media reform movement. The goals included limited ownership concentration in the media, increasing children's programming, requiring TV Stations to produce an hour of public affairs programming every evening, and reducing violence in programming.

Was it serendipitous or meant to be? Who knows? First, I am suddenly reconnected to that Nick Johnson who had urged me, and other classmates, to work in the public interest. Second, I had become fascinated with emerging digital technology. While on Capitol Hill, before joining the FTC, I had worked with the Commerce Committee staff, on behalf of Senator Durkin, on the emerging telephone (telecommunications) industry changes and new technologies. Although I was not and have never been an engineer and have no understanding of the technical side of new technologies, I did have the ability to understand or maybe sense the revolutionary impact that would emerge around new communications technology for consumers and society.

The opportunity was irresistible. It would be a big deal in Washington, DC, the consumer advocacy world, the communications industry, and indeed in Washington itself. All I had to do was persuade Susan that we could survive during a transition to an organization that had only $10,000 in the bank. Ralph and Nick were willing to commit to me a salary of $20,000. Of course, I would have to raise it, hopefully with their help.

This amounted to a different level of troublemaking for Susan and me. Going from a $150,000-a-year income to approximately $80,000 in gross salary, combining my $20,000 and Susan's $60,000, was disastrous. We started charging everything on our credit cards. When I took the helm at NCCB, there was one other staff person, a murky mission at the time, and little money in the bank.

I ultimately transformed the organization by changing its name to the Telecommunications Research and Action Center—known as TRAC—and its mission to represent consumer and public interests in the emerging telephone and telecommunication revolution.

It did very well for about nine years. We grew to nearly 20 staff members, published a monthly magazine, and I wrote several books. One, *Reverse the Charges, How to Save Money on Your Phone Bill*, published by Pantheon, was a Book-of-the-Month Club gift selection. (Well, they picked it as a "free" book if the customer bought the "Book-of-the-Month.")

In 1979, I served as the lawyer for dozens of consumers and non-profit groups in Washington, DC, before the judge in charge of breaking up AT&T. Yes, at one time, there was just one phone company—AT&T, which was declared a monopoly. The courts broke it into seven different regional phone companies. I was a major figure in that process as the lawyer representing multiple consumer groups.

My work was, once again, getting a lot of media attention. I didn't think anything would top that 1971 *New York Times* article, until now. I was on *Good Morning America*, January 1, 1984, the day the official breakup of AT&T went into effect. I was on the Phil Donahue Show when we wrote *Reverse the Charges*, and I was on the *Oprah Winfrey Show* when the "411" system was changed. Yes, by then, occasionally, someone in the grocery store would stare at me as if I were a celebrity.

Notwithstanding my high visibility, my low pay—I think my salary eventually increased to $25,000 a year—and the high expenses of living in McLean, Virginia, with two children kept us deep in debt. I remember the day when

Susan, who had always handled the day-to-day finances, came to me and "quit." She was crying and frustrated and almost yelled, "It's impossible. You do it and see if you can find the money to pay these bills."

It was a wake-up call. We had to make some changes. Besides enormous credit card debt, our two kids were approaching college age. We had no savings. We had to figure out what to do. The only solution was for me to find a way into the private sector.

My aha moment came when I realized I could serve as an intermediary between the growing telecommunications industry and the public interest groups I had represented. I founded a profitable public affairs company called Issue Dynamics, Inc. (IDI), with a vision to bridge the gap between industry and non-profit organizations and develop what I call "win-win" solutions.

I started small. It was just me with an idea and a desk in a borrowed office. From that small start, I created a nearly 50-person company that operated for about 25 years.

Over time, some of the newer, emerging advocates in the consumer arena became suspicious of me, some calling me a sellout for working so closely with the industry, who were, in fact, my clients. One advocate even created an entire website devoted to attacking me and trying to discredit my work. He portrayed me as Darth Vader, the evil man of the communications world. That didn't bother me or my clients. The bulk of the larger non-profits understood and valued the opportunity for meaningful interactions with the industry.

During this time, something important was happening that, in the end, defined the legacy of what I was able to accomplish. In the breakup of AT&T in 1979—the case where I was the "consumer attorney" representing these groups—one provision of the new law called for discounts to public education, schools, from the industry to enable them to purchase advanced telecommunication services such as high-speed internet services. Most school systems needed to rewire their entire networks, and the school buildings as well.

When it came time for the Federal Communications Commission (FCC) to write the regulations implementing this provision of the law, the phone companies, most of whom were my clients, said they wanted a plan that allowed them to provide discounts—something like 10 percent off the commercial/retail price. The non-profit groups, my friends, thought it was a scam concept. The phone company's "discount" was just a way for them to first jack the prices for the services by 15 percent, and then offer a 10 percent discount, they opined.

The schools had a different idea; they wanted actual money, cash, put into a new, advanced services fund administered by the FCC. It would be part of what is now known as the Universal Service Fund, or USF. The USF has been in existence for many years, designed to pay the cost of getting telephone services into high-cost or low-income areas of America. The FCC was experienced in granting funds upon applications by states and others. The consumer side, the folks I had worked with when I ran my non-profit group,

TRAC, wanted a similar system to be used for the new requirement to get advanced technology to schools.

The schools and the phone companies—who were nominally my clients, though they were paying me to work with the schools—were at a deadlock. The Federal Communications Commission was about to issue a decision. The schools knew the decision was going to be in their favor; the industry did too. Some in the industry were prepared to fight it out in the courts, which would delay the discounts for years and years, or maybe they would win and kill the plan entirely. One of my clients, one of the phone companies, thought I could help broker a compromise. Exactly my sweet spot in this business.

It was late on a Thursday. The FCC was going to meet the following Monday. The client called me and said his company wanted to present a new proposal for resolving this issue. Could I arrange for all the school stakeholders to meet with them the next day and hear them out?

Over the next few hours, I reached out to a dozen groups, including school unions and trade associations. I wasn't sure that I had either the credibility or the relationships to make something happen that quickly. I learned a profound lesson at that time. By building relationships with the groups over 20-plus years, with honesty and integrity, I had created a level of trust that enabled folks to take a risk, and they did.

It's a vivid moment, even now, so many years later. Everyone arrived on time and took a seat in a small conference room in our offices. About a dozen folks represented organizations like the National School Boards Association, the

National Education Association, the Association of School Principals, and a few others. There was a sole representative on behalf of most of the new regional telephone companies. Then there was me, the "go-between guy." I had everyone introduce themselves, and the industry guy laid out his idea. And then, silence.

Everyone just stared at each other. I wasn't certain what to do. I broke the silence with a plea to the school folks: "Say something, anything. You need to talk. That's why we are here." One of the education representatives, and a bit of a fan of mine at the time, asked a question. One simple question. That is all it took, and then boom, the dynamic in the room changed. Eventually, I stepped out of the room to allow the principals to do their deal, which was simple. Yes, the companies would put in cash to the Universal Service Fund, not offer so-called "discounts off rates," as long as the companies could put in the money "as it was needed." It simply meant a "pay-as-you-go plan" rather than a government-estimated number put up in advance. The agreement then needed to be vetted with a couple of the members of Congress who were closely following this issue. The FCC was informed of a "pending deal" and postponed its meeting for a day.

The agreement reached that day, and then cleared through members of the legislature, was presented to and adopted by the FCC. It became—and remains—the law. The amount deposited into the fund each year for the first few years was about two or three billion dollars. It has increased a few times since then. That was about 27 years or so ago, meaning that our work has resulted in about 50 billion dollars in funding for public schools to purchase and install "advanced technology services!"

I think now about that moment in time as an event and a result that justified the entire 25 years of my company. Sometimes, it takes 25 years to accomplish just one thing. Not only has the fund enabled schools all over the country to bring internet service to the classroom, something that today is considered routine if not necessary—but it has also helped bring internet services to rural and hard-to-reach areas.

As I write this in 2025, corporate power and influence are resurgent in America. Some industry players are challenging the funding framework we created back then. A New Orleans judge recently ruled that the Universal Service Fund itself—a fund created by the phone companies from their profits, and thus "ratepayer money"—is unconstitutional. The 5th Circuit Court of Appeals upheld that ruling. Just recently, the US Supreme Court reversed the decision and upheld the constitutionality of the Universal Service Fund. Historically, the Universal Service Fund was used to support access to basic phone services by low-income communities. Now, it is also being used to bring technology to islands of underserved consumers.

We also used a similar technique to get another change in the law. Working with the disability community, we organized a coalition to collaborate with the telephone industry and together convince Congress to require that new (advanced) technology—digital communication services, referred to as "advanced services" in the law—be developed and offered in ways accessible to people with disabilities. It continues to be the law of the land.

Indeed, as I am writing and living with a neurocognitive disability, others and I in the disability community are working under the Americans with Disability Act, rather than the Communications law, so that the newer technologies can be accessible to folks like us.

The financial success of Issue Dynamics allowed me to pay off all those credit card bills and get my kids through college. It also allowed us to travel a lot. I opened an office for my company in San Francisco. Two important things happened on the West Coast.

First, I was asked to serve on the board of directors of the World Institute on Disability (WID), headquartered in Oakland, California, right across the Bay from what was then Issue Dynamics, Inc, San Francisco office. Second, it allowed me to travel and meet a relative living in Seattle, Washington. At WID, I worked with folks like the late Judy Heumann, who had become known as the mother of modern disability policy. I also got to work with the late Professor Frank Bowe, who was a professor at Hofstra University. Frank worked with me in Washington, DC, as a consultant to IDI and eventually became known as the father of the modern disability movement.

At the time, I didn't have a disability—well, I didn't think I had a disability. WID's rules allowed only a small proportion of the board to be people without a known disability. I don't know why I was moved to be so active in disability rights. It might have been that my sister Harriet, as I've mentioned, had a cognitive disorder and was diagnosed with "Low IQ" later in life. Or maybe my interest or empathy was because my one "disorder" was terrible handwriting, and I was often ridiculed for it. Or maybe there really is a troublemaker gene that we haven't discovered yet, and I needed to be a troublemaker for more accessibility. Somehow, I just "got it" and eventually was vice-chair of the Board of Directors of WID.

The work with WID and the engagement, as a result, with the larger disability movement in the United States has become an enormously valuable asset for me as I face Alzheimer's dementia. I now have real-world models of individuals who have challenges, both physical and cognitive, who do live fully engaged in the larger world, with whatever accommodations facilitate that outcome. On reflection, I think my exposure to people who lived with an array of significant disabilities—deaf, blind, intellectual, physical (movement), breathing, and more—who still were able to run the organization and live meaningful and productive lives, has allowed me to imagine that even with Alzheimer's I, too, can lead an active and fruitful life.

Many of those people have become lifelong friends. I instinctively understood—and that understanding was reaffirmed in my engagement with the WID staff—that despite their differences, people with disabilities have a right to an independent, meaningful life, with agency and choices. Every human being has the potential to contribute to our community. The time I spent working extensively within the disability movement has, I am sure, shaped my perspective today as I enter that community. Once again, I look back at events and activities in my life over decades that seemed to have enabled my future. It's as if fate, an unknown force, knew what would happen to me and prepared me for even this Alzheimer's journey.

Indeed, today, I am a man with a cognitive disability who is losing his cognitive capacity to function normally in the world. Thanks in a very large part to my time on the Board of WID, I have been privileged to see, meet, and work with people with severe physical and cognitive disabilities. My inspiration and beliefs today come in significant part from my time at WID.

We have miles to go yet, though, for those of us with neurocognitive disorders stemming from various brain diseases or other cognitive disorders. Indeed, the historic narrative in America, and the world, has been that life with neurocognitive disorders—aka dementia—is not worth living. History, as I understand it, has carried with it a grand tragedy narrative, and a "why me" mindset.

It was the world I thought I was going to step into as I was coming to terms with my diagnosis of Alzheimer's disease. I would hear and read the voices of those choosing to end their own life rather than choosing to live the best lives possible until the end. Even now, as I write this book and take my journey, I read obituaries of those, occasionally some folks I know, who went to Switzerland for suicide. There are competing advocacy organizations, those opposing accompanied suicide, and those supporting "the right to die" or "assisted suicide."

I am not a superhero nor a superman. I am just someone whose life journey seems to have been set before me to prepare me for just this moment, the beginning of my final journey. Yes, I choose life.

CHAPTER 9

SUSAN'S EXISTENTIAL JOURNEY

Twenty-five years or so ago, there was a dress rehearsal for what I am facing today. I mentioned it earlier: Susan's breast cancer, the doctors' finding an unexpected post-mastectomy lump, and pulling me aside and whispering, "Get ready." That moment lives with me today as bright and deep inside me as the moment it happened. Indeed, my purpose here is to note—perhaps honor—that experience because it is, I believe, what gives me today the strength and focus to do my Alzheimer's differently.

Susan had worked on and off during the first decade or so of our marriage. She was a stay-at-home mom of our children until they were old enough for childcare, and then headed back into the work force. By the time we lived in Northern Virginia, 1970, she had earned a master's degree in special education. Years later, she became certified as an elementary school counselor in the grade school system. After retirement as a teacher, she returned to school to receive a certification in the field of eldercare. She and a friend decided to start a new business, consulting with families whose loved ones needed care. I was excited for her, and I had registered the name: "Elder Affairs." I loved the double entendre!

Throughout this latter part of her career, in the Northern Virginia area, I was the CEO of my company, Issue Dynamics. It was in about the 20th year or so of IDI when Susan's diagnosis with breast cancer disrupted our lives. As mentioned previously, this entire episode of our lives became my first play and is documented in a stand-alone book by the same name, *The Actual Dance, Love's Ultimate Journey Through Breast Cancer.*

Susan's treatment included a radical double mastectomy. Back then, the mastectomy was performed before the patient (Susan in this case) was seen by an oncologist. So, Susan's first appointment with her oncologist happened about six weeks after the double mastectomy. It was also after the hospital admitted that they had made a mistake and that there was significant cancer found in many of Susan's lymph nodes.

In some ways, our journey in the early 2000s became a dress rehearsal for my journey 18 years later. In Susan's case, we arrive together for that first appointment with her oncologist. At this point, Susan had largely recovered from her double mastectomy and the removal of 11 cancerous lymph nodes. The goal of an oncologist appointment is to come up with a post-surgery treatment plan, presumably chemotherapy and radiation therapy. The doctor's first step is to examine the surgical area where the breasts had been.

Given our history so far of misdiagnosis, I insist on being in the room for this examination. I can be a second set of eyes and ears, and a cross-examiner if needed. I watch as the oncologist has Susan take off her blouse. The nurse unwraps the bandage still covering the scar lines of the mastectomy. Susan then lies down on the exam table.

I stand back and watch the doctor put his hands on Susan's now scarred, bare upper chest. It is briefly odd, for me, to see another man's hands on her bare chest. His fingers go from the right toward the left side of her chest, where the breasts had been, sliding along the scar line. Before reaching the opposite end, he abruptly stops. He stands straight up, as if at attention, does a military-style about-face, marches past me to the other side of the room, and picks up the phone. It turns out he's found a post-mastectomy lump on Susan's chest. He is calling her breast surgeon to tell him about the lump and to schedule an urgent appointment.

The breast surgeon juggles his schedule and sees Susan the next day. He can also feel the lump and immediately schedules her for surgery to remove it. Neither the oncologist nor the breast surgeon says it out loud, though it is clear to me, based on their demeanor, that she—indeed, we—need to get ready for an inevitable bad ending.

As you have read, Susan and I had become familiar with end-of-life experiences by that time in our lives. Susan's mother and father, my father and mother, one of my sisters, and numerous aunts and uncles had passed. So, death was no stranger, and the rituals around the end of life were familiar. Yet it had never been about us.

It is the beginning of a transformative period of our lives. Each of us is affected in very different ways: ways now, in retrospect, that seemed to have sharpened the edges of who we were from deep within our being. Confronting the mortality of ourselves—or our life partner—awakens each of us to life and purpose in radically meaningful ways.

During the nearly three years of Susan's active treatment, my role in life transforms from that of a successful businessman, expanding his business and growing his profile in Washington, DC, to that of Susan's care partner. I prefer "LovePartner™." My priority shifts from maintaining the growth and success of my company, Issue Dynamics, Inc., to doing everything I can to be a comforting partner for Susan throughout what seems to be her final stage of life.

I still remember sitting down with each of the nearly 50 employees at Issue Dynamics to tell them my situation and that I would be out of the office a lot. My vice president, Ken, takes over much of the responsibility for managing daily activities.

I start spending the nights in the hospital with Susan, sleeping on a cot next to her bed. During that time, I get used to helping her get out of bed with all those infusion lines in her veins and walk to the bathroom. When she gets nauseous from the chemotherapy drugs, I hold that semi-circular metal pan in front of her when she vomits. Things in the normal course of my life to that date, I have somehow managed to avoid.

The anticipated loss of Susan, wife and mother, triggers significant changes in all daily life routines. For me, of course, as I have described. And now in the lives of our two grown children.

Our son was about to start his three-year tour of active duty in the US Army Judge Advocate General Corps. Yes, he was following in my footsteps. Marcus and his wife were excited. Early in their marriage, with no children, they secured an assignment in South Korea. They planned to spend two of their three-year active-duty commitment there, and then a year somewhere else. Instead, given his mother's illness, our son asks and receives a compassionate change in deployment so he can serve his active duty near his mom. They spend all three years of their active-duty commitment in Northern Virginia.

Stationed in Northern Virginia, much like Susan and I did when I was in the Army in Fort Lee, Virginia, they, too, manage to purchase a home. It's located near where we live. It is hard to know what would have happened if they had gone to Korea. What did happen is that they became deeply embedded in our community, and they built incredible connections that serve them both well.

At that time, our daughter was a newly minted pediatric dentist working in an office near Baltimore, Maryland. As her practice permits, she finds a way to squeeze in time off to visit us and spend time with her mom. The drive from her home near Baltimore, Maryland, and McLean, Virginia, takes anywhere from thirty minutes to more than an hour each way, depending on traffic. She also serves as an informal medical sounding board as I try to deepen my understanding of the medical jargon and changes in Susan's health. She continues in that role today, as we navigate Alzheimer's disease. We ask a lot of questions, and she keeps reminding us she is a dentist, not a cancer doctor.

My life, too, is uprooted and transformed during that time. The prospect of losing Susan in what seems the prime of our marriage and our lives is profound, emotional, and disorienting. Those words seem inadequate, because by the end of this experience, I have become a different person. During the process, as Susan's prognosis becomes grimmer, I begin to understand my responsibility. I will have to hold her, be with her, comfort her, and assure her that there is an eternal place of ecstatic goodness, and I will hold her as she leaves me for that place. I experience a sense of inevitability and certainty that I cannot share with anyone, not even Susan.

As Susan and I wait for the procedure to remove and then analyze the lump, the post-double-mastectomy lump, Susan is stoic. Like a rock. She insists that anyone in her presence be positive and not show anxiety or fear. The only way for me to do that is to bury that fear and put it deep inside.

In fact, in retrospect, it was an experience in some way not unlike my experiences now with what I call "The Nothingness Place." It seems that I have this ability to transform during existential moments in my life, literally experiencing a different dimension of existence.

With Susan, there were moments when I would exit the "real world" and travel to into a liminal place between "here"—the world—and "there"—a waystation on the journey to the end—death. There, Susan and I would join together, embracing, as she would take her last breath. I would be holding her, we would be in a ballroom, and the music of hearts (Unchained Melody) would be playing, as her life exited into eternity.

My understanding has evolved since that time. I have come to think of that experience as a form of Post-Traumatic Spiritual Disorder. Just as Susan was displaying stoic commitment to "beat this thing," externally, I was too. Internally, something different was happening. It was a sense of me, my spirit, if not my body, leaving this world, an existential exit from the earthly bonds. Clearly, not our physical bodies—rather, our spiritual bodies—there in a liminal place, perhaps a parallel spiritual universe, where we would dance.

The experience years ago changed me and shaped my soul. It taught me what love really means. As difficult as it was then, it has become a blessing for today, as Susan and I have changed places. It has informed both of us of our unique roles with each other—to be a reciprocal strength. To share ourselves without question or fear.

I am convinced there has been a divine hand, sometimes thought of as Grace, helping us in our lives. Susan's surprise turn in her career, from being a grade-school counselor to working in the aging field, has prepared her for this next dramatic turn in our lives. Sam has Alzheimer's.

Now, it is my "turn at the wheel," so to speak. We have pivoted from my service as her care partner as we anticipated her death from breast cancer to Susan now being my care partner following my diagnosis of Alzheimer's, which, as of 2025, is a non-curable condition.

I do not yet have the language or conceptual framework to explain how I feel blessed and lucky to be in this relationship with Susan, and this journey we are on. It isn't about what we wanted or would have chosen; it is about what has happened and the ability to experience the love of the other in these existential engagements.

Perhaps the life lesson for us, Susan and me, in these events is the discovery of how to live meaningful and whole lives with whatever happens. I would never have wanted Susan to have gone through that breast cancer experience. Her near-death experience oddly changed me more than her. It touched me to my core and provided fundamental insights into love and life. Ultimately, I was led to an entirely new life and career. I found my way into theatre, playwriting, and performance. This fourth age, as I call it, has been a multi-step process, and it is not yet over.

I have learned that in a marriage or a relationship, while there are indeed two physical people, each unique, a new entity can arise: A singularity consisting of what had been two and is now a single, interconnected soul. In the context of Susan and me, I have eventually come to call the entity: *US*. I wrote a poem by that name:

> *US*
> *Life exists within each of us as a form of the Divine*
> *A tangible essence of who we are.*

Love is when our essence becomes entwined
Each an equal half of the other.
"I love you" awakens the US in you and me.
I Love You.

Our experience of Susan's near-death, and the process of coming to terms with that experience, resulted in a profound transformation of our relationship. Susan and I then entered a period of nearly twenty years of health, joy, and meaning.

Yes, Susan's experience of being near death was a form of a dress rehearsal for what we are going through now. Susan and I have discovered new levels of deep intimacy, both physical and spiritual intimacy—lessons to us of what love means. I wonder occasionally if the experience with Susan almost dying was necessary training for both of us to deal with this moment in our journey.

It is me—Sam Simon—who now has a terminal diagnosis.

CHAPTER 10

THE ALZHEIMER'S DIAGNOSIS
STARTING MY EXISTENTIAL JOURNEY

So, yes, Dr. Howard just gave me the prescription for Aricept and abruptly walked out of the room, without providing instructions, and never attempted to contact me after that appointment. We didn't care at that point because Susan and I already understood we needed to find a new doctor.

Susan and I booked that appointment with Dr. Banks, the referral from our gym friend Ellen. The six weeks it takes to see him soon becomes the norm for us in this neurological world. As the boomer generation is heading into their eighth decade, the medical world seems overwhelmed with the explosion of cognitive disorders.

In 2025, we seem to be on the edge of an explosion in new treatments and drugs for cognitive disorders and especially Alzheimer's. Yet, for most of modernity, dementia or mental disorders have been seen as unmentionable tragedies, echoing the early culture and fears around cancer. There was a time when the word "cancer" could not be said in polite company. It was "the C word." Indeed, the brain is perhaps the most mysterious organ of all.

As we wait to see Dr. Banks, our experience with the first neurologist, Dr. Howard, weighs heavily on us. Would this be the same? Would his style be any better? Could he offer us some hope for a meaningful future? So, our entry into the office of the new neurologist is tentative. We don't know what to think or what to expect.

The experience is radically different—night and day, if we want a trite expression. First, when we enter the treatment room for that first appointment after filling out all the routine paperwork, he is waiting for us. He is not rushed in his approach. He is welcoming and interested in us. Where are we from? What brought us to him? Susan and I discuss our family and careers.

He begins by explaining that he has reviewed the neuropsychologist's report and that he agrees with the diagnosis of Mild Cognitive Impairment (MCI). Unlike Dr. Howard, he doesn't get up and leave the room. He continues. The next necessary step is to get to the bottom of why I am impaired and to come up with a treatment plan. Susan and I look at each other, with the knowing look that says: "Yes, that's why we are here!"

Dr. Banks says the only way to know what's going on with me for sure is to get a PET/CT with contrast. It is the gold standard for determining the cause of cognitive impairment. The test costs thousands of dollars and, at the time, was typically not covered by insurance. Today, that is beginning to change somewhat, driven, in part, by the growing number of dementia cases within the Baby Boom cohort.

Dr. Howard had brought up the PET/CT and blew it off as too expensive in a way that made it seem that the test was not that important.

It turns out we were confused about more than just that.

Dr. Howard had told us that the MRI I'd had didn't reveal any black tangles, a condition caused by a variant of the tau protein of the brain that has been abnormally modified. Of course, he was right. The MRI didn't show that because, we have since learned, MRIs don't detect tau—PET/CT scans with contrast do. As noted above, Dr. Howard had mentioned the latter in passing but didn't suggest I have one. The MRI simply showed that the "shrinkage" of my brain was normal for a man my age.

Dr. Howard also neglected to address amyloid plaques, another indication of Alzheimer's. We now know that to diagnose a person with Alzheimer's disease, the doctor needs to ascertain whether they have either amyloid plaques or those tau protein tangles. Dr. Howard tested for neither.

Now, in this visit, after confirming the MCI and the need for the scan, Dr. Banks proposes a workaround for us to avoid the costs of the PET/CT. He explains that he is friends with a Dr. Scott, the neurologist who leads the University Memory Center in the neurology department of a large Washington, DC, hospital. The Center does treat patients, though their main work has evolved into hosting trials for new drugs related to cognition. With my diagnosis of MCI, I could be a candidate for one of those drug trials.

First, though, the University Medical Center will need to know as much about my condition as possible, which means, if accepted, I would get one of those fancy PET/CT scans with contrast to determine if I qualify. Well, as it turns out, I arrive at Dr. Scott's program at just the right time. The Memory Center had just received a US government grant to create a "trial-ready cohort." That meant the US government would pay for the full testing of people with cognitive problems to determine if they are potential candidates for the growing number of clinical trials of new drugs being brought to market. Those tests include both MRIs and the PET/CT with contrast. First, though, I am required to go through all the other standard cognitive tests once again. These big, fancy neurology programs at universities doing drug trials don't accept anyone else's test results. Therefore, I need to endure yet another series of studies that resemble the earlier neuropsychological studies, though not precisely the same.

Susan and I show up at what is a very large hospital complex. Everything is unfamiliar, which adds emotional weight to our experiences. We struggle to find the right floor, check in, and then fill out all sorts of forms. Susan and I would typically be invited into a nurse's or doctor's office for an initial interview.

This time, something new. The first step is for Susan and me to be interviewed by a neuropsychologist—separately. We immediately get split up and taken in opposite directions with our own interviewers. I am surprised and confused. I get agitated. "Why is Susan being interviewed? No one else has interviewed her."

No one explains the process in advance, which we now know is routine. They want to learn from my wife, who is now identified as my caregiver, about what she sees in me on a day-to-day basis. What is she observing? This process becomes evident to us once we are involved in it.

Without me in the room, Susan is asked how she thinks I am doing. Next, she is asked to recount, with details, something that has happened recently involving both of us—a story of sorts. Of course, they also ask her about her observations on changes in me, and my ability to perform daily tasks.

The interviews last all morning. When we break for lunch, Susan and I are escorted into what was once a hospital room. It is now an empty room with a bed and a small table. We sit down at the table, scrunched in a corner, as lunch is brought to us. As soon as we are alone, I grill her. Frustrated and probably sounding angry, I bark, "What did they ask you about me? What did you tell them? Why are they talking to you?" She tells me she isn't allowed to talk about it. That frustrated me even more.

We stop talking to each other until the person who interviewed Susan in the morning shows up to interview me. Again, something that will become standard practice in the future, although a surprise at the time. Having asked Susan for a story about something that happened in our lives, the interviewer now asks me about the story, to see what I remember. In this case, it goes like this:

"Sam, Susan told me about a trip you two took this past weekend. She mentioned that you stopped somewhere on the way, perhaps for lunch. What do you remember?"

I close my eyes and think: "A trip. Did we take a trip? No, we didn't take a *trip*! Oh, wait, yes, we went to LodgeBend." (This is the name we have given to our second home.) "That isn't a trip, is it? Oh, I guess it is, and I do remember going there. Yes, I remember, but when? Was it last weekend or two weeks ago?" I wonder if this is a trick question. I think, and think, and then it occurs to me, "Yes, it was last weekend! Stop for lunch? No. We always do a bathroom stop. Susan almost always needs to stop for a potty break. She can't hold it, I could, but if we stop, as we typically do, I take advantage of it. A bathroom stop. Yes! Not lunch though."

The next moments are confusing as I try to recall a trip and go through all those disjointed thoughts. I have no recollection of verbally responding to the interviewer. It seems as if I am still looking for the answer, with my eyes closed, and then being woken up by the interviewer saying rather loudly, "Time's up! You did well, Sam." I don't remember saying anything.

It takes six weeks after that appointment for us to receive the results from the Memory Center and obtain a third confirming opinion. Yes, they agree, freshly tested, not just looking at the results from my previous doctor, I am Mildly Cognitively Impaired. As a result, I am eligible for the PET/CT with contrast. That is the third confirming opinion. Dr. Howard, Dr. Banks, and now the University Memory Center.

Being eligible doesn't get me the scan by itself. Instead, it throws me into a whole new process and additional qualifying exams. It takes six weeks to initiate the process, which includes a first appointment with a different department. Another six weeks for the testing, then I am told I qualify, and I get that cherished PET/CT with contrast. Of course, it takes another six weeks for the test results to come in, and they are not sent to us. Rather, they are sent to Dr. Banks. Yes, it winds up being 18 weeks, a little more than four months to get through the process.

We call Dr. Banks' office to set an appointment to get the results, which takes another three weeks. In retrospect, the fact that it took only three weeks, not the typical six weeks, probably should have been a hint that something was up.

This next appointment is different. We are not taken to an examination room this time. Instead, as soon as we walk into the office suite, a person emerges from behind the registration desk and says, "Follow me." She guides us down a long hallway, past the doors to the treatment rooms, stops in front of Dr. Banks's private office, and knocks on the door. We hear Dr. Bank's voice, "Enter." As the door opens, Dr. Banks doesn't look up; he gestures for us to enter.

Dr. Banks sits behind his desk, a large brown folder on his lap, showing a smaller vanilla folder with a single sheet of white paper sticking out. He seems reserved as he motions us towards two chairs across from his desk. There is no eye contact. He looks down at the paper.

"I think we are at a new diagnosis." He pauses, looks down again, and then mumbles, "Early-stage Alzheimer's disease."

It seems odd to me now, looking back on the experience. As his last words— "Alzheimer's disease"—are leaving his mouth, there begins an infinite moment when the universe itself seems to stop. The room is silent. He lets the moment sit, as do we all. The three of us in the room just sit, we don't react. Susan and I can sense that this is bad news, and yet we don't ask him why or what it means. We simply capture the moment.

Having gone through this process before regarding Susan's seemingly relentless bad-news breast cancer experience, I know now that giving very bad news is also hard for many doctors. Some simply imply it and allow the patient to figure it out. After all, today, there is Doctor Google.

I think Dr. Banks is trying to be the best possible deliverer of medically terrible news. We can tell he is very uncomfortable. Indeed, his body and tone communicate that this is bad news. We know that Alzheimer's is not curable. So does he. Yet neither he nor we spend any time focusing on that fact.

When Dr. Banks finally speaks again, he seeks to give us a vision of the journey forward that holds some hope. He tells us that it could take five to ten years for the symptoms to get a lot worse. I don't know if he means five to ten years from the date of diagnosis in 2022 or five to ten years from the onset of the disease. A date which is not marked anywhere. What does "start" mean anyway, with Alzheimer's? Perhaps from when I started showing symptoms? Was that way back when I complained to my previous internist about my memory, and then could not remember what I had for breakfast that day? Or was it when I started driving on the wrong side of the road?

It takes a little bit of time for us—Susan and me—to absorb the diagnosis. Alzheimer's is worse than cancer. There are long-term survivors of many cancers. In fact, "cured" is in cancer vocabulary. Susan is here today, 26 years after her diagnosis of what the doctors then thought was going to be terminal. She is the outlier. There are no outliers of Alzheimer's disease yet.

It is possible, though, that as someone diagnosed later in life—I am 77 at that point—my end-of-life might be the result of some other condition. Indeed, while writing this book, I have been diagnosed with early-stage prostate cancer. After analysis, my urologist recommended "watchful waiting." At my age, it is not expected that cancer will have time to spread before something else gets me. Even if it does start to spread, several treatments will slow, if not stop, its spread and, indeed, cure me. Indeed, as I write this, the urologist has told me they have now discovered cells in my urine that are strong indicators of bladder cancer. The urologist, however, can't find it, so various new tests are being conducted to locate what he believes is an emerging cancer elsewhere. Yet, unlike with Alzheimer's, there can be a cure for whatever cancer they might find.

In either case, even as I write this, I am not ready to die. I still have work to do. I want to be married to Susan for 60 or 70 or even more years. Yes, I want a diamond anniversary—75th! Just 18 more years from now. Okay, I know that isn't likely, even if I didn't have Alzheimer's or prostate cancer—I would be 96 at that point. Do I harbor dreams of beating all odds? Why not! At least I want to try.

I want to see my oldest granddaughter, Emily, grow up and become a Jewish professional or whatever she truly wants to be. Yes, I'm a typical Jewish grandfather. Susan and I are committed to our Jewish faith and are deeply involved in our Reform Jewish synagogue, Temple Rodef Shalom, in Falls Church, Virginia. We have modeled to our children what a committed Jewish life is like today, and then some. Susan and I have each served a term as president of our congregation, which is now one of the largest Reform synagogues in America.

Emily is 23 years old as I write this. She graduated from the University of Delaware with her Bachelor of Arts in Political Science in May 2025. She is pursuing a master's degree in public administration and is expected to receive her Master of Arts in Public Administration in 2026.

We have two other granddaughters, children of our daughter, Rachael Simon. That is Dr. Rachael Simon, a pediatric dentist. Rachael has kept her birth last name for professional use in her pediatric practice. Her husband is David Proper, and she uses Rachael Proper in family settings.

Her two children are a bit younger than Emily. As I write this, Sydney will be 17 soon and is a senior in high school (she graduated in May 2025). Based on her lacrosse skills and good grades, she has already received a full four-year scholarship to college in Pennsylvania. Her goal is to become a physical therapist, and the college she will attend has a physical therapy graduate program, with a spot for her if she maintains a good grade point average. She has been a lacrosse goalie throughout middle and high school, and she is good. She has already traveled to Israel to practice with Israel's national women's lacrosse team as part of a program to connect Israeli and American talent.

Her younger sister, Joanna, whom we call JoJo, is about to become a junior in high school. She is also sports-oriented and has served a period as captain of one of the school volleyball teams. She is also running track. JoJo had a time when she seemed interested in becoming a dancer. I could imagine her as Gypsy Rose Lee on Broadway. She loves to dance and move. She is artistic and has a good voice. Oh, and she had a fascination with unicorns for a while.

JoJo and Sydney are also very active in Jewish youth groups like their cousin Emily was when she was in high school.

Then there is our only grandson, Zachary, Emily's younger brother. As I write this, he is starting his sophomore year in college. Virginia Tech is the same college where his mother spent four years. Zach has played every sport there is through high school, except contact football. His mom would not let him do that. He is charting a course of his own. Early on, Zach didn't seem interested in Jewish life. His mom is now on the executive board of the temple and might one day be the third Simon to be President of the congregation. It wasn't until Zach spent a semester in Israel that he developed an interest in Judaism and connecting with other Jewish kids.

Zach is indeed coming out of his shell. I learned recently that he is an emerging leader in his fraternity, and the Jewish Council of the University. He is considering running for president of the council. Maybe he will be like his dad and become a politician!

I don't know what they will become. I want to be around to see what happens for all our grandchildren and maybe even great-grandchildren one day. I want to watch the future generations grow and continue the legacy of the Sam and Susan Simon family. Celebrate from generation to generation.

Isn't that what we all want?

We don't always get what we want, do we?

When Susan and I get home after hearing the news that I have Alzheimer's disease, we arrange for a Zoom call with our children, Marcus and Rachael. We don't want to include our son-in-law or daughter-in-law in these things yet. It's hard to know what the right thing to do is. We are the ones who are supposed to know, right? And yet at these existential moments, it's like being in a dark room looking for an exit.

On Zoom, our adult children, both now in their 50s, are calm and offer reassuring and loving support. There are no answers, no effort to tell us what to do, and no asking us what we plan to do.

The following two steps seem obvious. One is an appointment with our estate attorney. When we call to set the appointment, he says we should have our children present and that the "kids" should be involved in whatever plan we come up with.

Next, I must notify our temple's senior rabbi and cantor. I suspect it is often a first thought for people to send a message to their priest or rabbi when they get a terminal diagnosis. After all, it is an "existential moment." What's religion about if it isn't life and death and the meaning of life and death?

I get a call back from each, and the cantor invites me to lunch. It turns out his mother and father have had forms of cognitive decline, aka dementia. He gives me advice, including suggestions on getting my affairs in order and thinking about where to relocate when I need to be elsewhere. The thoughts prove helpful, and we have begun looking into future housing options.

We, Susan and I, understand the road that I am on with great clarity. At moments, my sense of getting worse, my vanishing into and out of nothingness, is screaming at me: "Decide, Sam. Your time is running out. You have to decide now!"

Indeed, if I were to want to go to Switzerland for accompanied suicide, I would need to decide very soon. One must be mentally "competent" to give "informed consent." In other words, I would have to be judged sane or competent by a licensed mental health professional to be allowed to go down that path. I am acutely aware that things can change quickly and unexpectedly. Maybe the next time I dissolve into nothingness, I won't come out.

I am reminded of the phenomenon that occurs after buying a new vehicle and then noticing all the cars on the road that are the same type or color as our newly purchased car. It seems that it happens to everyone. Buy a new Jeep, and suddenly it seems like Jeeps are everywhere. We bought a bright blue Toyota Rav4 once, and I remember how many bright blue cars we noticed. It seems, too, that now that I must confront what to do next, I am reading and hearing about so many people who have chosen the accompanied-suicide route.

While writing this book, I came across an obituary in *The Washington Post* for Hal Malchow, a Washington, DC, political analyst. Hal was a well-known name in Democratic circles for some time, and I am sure that I worked with or around him during my career. Hal had opted for Switzerland, accompanied suicide. He was 72. His obituary reads like the identical story of my journey. He had Alzheimer's, and earlier this year—that means the last three months—he also wrote and published a book. Reading that obituary raises the stakes for me. What should I do?

So, if I want to take the trip to Switzerland, Susan and I had better start the process.

It is an existential question: When is life worth living? Perhaps more accurately, when is life NOT worth living? What if I have another five, even ten, reasonably productive years ahead of me? Maybe part of my getting worse is an equal part disease and an equal part normal aging? If I can't tell and want to go to Switzerland, then there is urgency in making the plans and getting it done.

Yet, in many ways, my current symptoms are insignificant. Apart from those moments in The Nothingness Place, I can lead a decent life, and the more accommodations that become available, the more I can enjoy life. There are new therapies, new medicines. Who knows how much we can slow the march of this lumbering disease?

It occurs to me, too, that for those who do not want to go through the worst parts of the end, there is another option. I wonder why folks like Hal Malchow do not wait until they sense the end is imminent, and if they still want to end it, then commit suicide. Live for as long as we can, as productively as possible, then just end our own lives.

So, I can wait and experience as much of a full and meaningful life as possible, despite being a deeply forgetful person. Continue to perform my play, finish this book, tell my story, and become a leader in the movement to change how the world sees us "people with dementia." Get into a new drug trial, or just be alert, aware of my condition, even as I decline. See all my grandchildren grow up, and maybe even meet a great-grandchild! Only when I begin to sense that I am approaching the very end of that long, dark decline into loss of identity and personhood—about to fold up and disappear, or change, or become too impaired to function at home or in a meaningful way—I could then just kill myself. I don't need to be "mentally competent" to do that.

I just need to have the capacity to time it right. Make sure I will still be able to operate a car and figure things out. It would be easy to make the short drive from our McLean, Virginia, home to the Chain Bridge, which spans the Potomac River just north of the Georgetown area of Washington, DC. The irony is that we live right off Chain Bridge Road, which goes from McLean to the bridge. Making the short, three-mile trip to the Chain Bridge would be a snap. I could park the car right at the edge of the bridge as it starts to leave Virginia. Get out and walk 100 feet or so to the middle of the bridge, and, assuming I have the guts, jump into the Potomac River.

The topic of what to do never seems to go away for me, and I wonder, too, about my family. No one tells me they want me dead. Susan is committed to be my LovePartner™—to be with me through the end. We don't talk out loud about it that much because we both still know that we are "*US.*" A singularity, a shared soul. Well, that isn't exactly true, because even as I write this book, my cognitive capacity is changing. My inability to recall, often insisting that I'm right and she's wrong, can explode into mini shouting matches. I can tell it is hard for her sometimes. She is stoic. I don't know how to interpret stoicism, because I can't see to the other side of it.

Yes, the topic of suicide does come up from time to time, like that morning I opened the newspaper and read the obituary of Hal Malchow. Why didn't Hal wait longer?

It comes up when I listen to a podcast about a book, with the author bragging about how she helped her husband kill himself.

It comes up when I get frustrated with simple tasks in life, such as finding my toothpaste or paying bills online.

Every time I have a doctor's appointment because at the end of each appointment, there is the familiar ritual of asking if I have ever had suicidal thoughts.

The questions on those forms: *Have you ever considered killing yourself? Have you ever thought about committing suicide? Have you ever started to hurt yourself and then stopped? Have you ever started to hurt yourself, and someone else stopped you?* I still answer, "No."

I wonder if anyone, especially people who do kill themselves, ever answered "Yes."

CHAPTER 11

WHAT TO DO NOW?

It is now mid-2025, about five years after that visit with Dr. Banks, when he delivered the diagnosis of Alzheimer's disease and said it could take five to ten years before things started to get a lot worse. In fact, it is seven years after my diagnosis of Mild Cognitive Impairment, which is perhaps when my disease started to get worse. At our most recent appointment, a few days ago, I mentioned to him that I was feeling that things are deteriorating. More memory glitches— they feel different, and my cognition seems more compromised. He doesn't try to minimize it; he doesn't ask questions. Instead, in a sort of "I told you so" tone of voice, he says, "Yes, it is getting worse," or words to that effect. Oddly, his tone surprises me. I was hoping he would have been more reassuring.

My questions about what to do next started shortly after I was diagnosed with Mild Cognitive Impairment in 2018 and continue to this day. Life seems to operate simultaneously in the present, past, and future. That initial phase was a time, in many ways, much like today, though less intense. My life was truly blessed, and I was determined that this memory thing wouldn't spoil it, if I could help it. Theater and art were overtaking my social justice journey. My play, *The Actual Dance: Love's Ultimate Journey Through Breast Cancer,* was getting great notice, and I performed frequently. I spoke, to a world I had not known about, the emotional journey of the caregiver, or care partner or, my term for the journey: *LovePartner*™. Over the course of about a ten-year period, I learned how to produce it, which involved securing bookings and funding. Luckily, I received financial support from the Collegiate Church and Emblem Health, a major insurance company in New York that had a significant program supporting family caregivers.

In the fifth year of performing that play, in January 2019, I returned to the national conference of the Association of Performing Arts Professionals, also known as APAP, in New York City, which I had been attending for several years. It was initially the trade association of American presenting theaters—think Kennedy Center, Carnegie Hall, and all the local regional stages or stages in the colleges near you. They all go to New York in January to compare experiences as "presenters" and to peruse new works.

Sam Simon and his one-man show at APAP is like a sentence in a thousand-page book. There are hundreds of agents pitching their clients to these theaters. Three floors of booths, mainly pitching the traveling theatrical shows, comedians, musicians, singers, performing well-known classic pieces, and musicians playing all genres of music. Dancers and ballets. Mostly, though, their theatrical agents—yes, three full floors of people, tables, the echoing "Book me," "Book my client," etc. Then there is little me, Sam Simon, and his one-man play. Well, I'm just this guy who has written a one-man show.

At my first conference, I was given sage counsel by several seasoned attendees that I have since learned to be true: there are many folks like me—young, naïve, first-time attendees with new work—out there in the theater world. Actors and playwrights with new work who think that if we show up once at APAP, the theater world will be astonished and see us as the "new big thing." Why wouldn't they? We have so much good feedback from our homies and friends.

"Sam, you need to come back to this conference over and over and over again," I was told. "Develop personal relationships with presenters and agents. Establish a reputation as a professional in the field and establish that you are in the game for the long haul." That was hard to hear. Of course, I also needed a good product with its own history of production. I took that advice to heart. My attendance in 2025 was my tenth year (counting the two years of remote events during the pandemic).

I had one other piece of good luck, besides that good advice that I followed. At one of the regional theater conferences, I met a theatrical agent named Milt Orkin during a coffee break between sessions while I was walking from table to table, introducing myself and handing out literature. Milt was kind and took my materials, and when he realized it was about my wife having breast cancer. He immediately perked up. His wife was just finishing her breast-cancer journey. We connected after the conference, and he got permission from his agency to bring me on as a client. Having a theatrical agent listed on my materials skyrocketed my credibility. A confirmation for me that my job, my task is to just show up.

By 2018, I had become a known quantity among many at APAP. I remember the shift, the turn of my reputation. One individual, a well-known and highly respected magician/actor, had typically given me a hard time, along with some of the other new performers at earlier APAP conferences. As I entered the exhibit hall at the 2018 APAP event, and walked past this fellow's booth, he stopped me and said, "Hey Sam, I am hearing a lot of good stuff about your show!"

Then, in January 2019, worried about my MCI, I needed to decide what to do. I started talking to my colleagues and now trusted fellow theatre producers, tentatively at first. I didn't know much about cognitive impairment myself. "I don't know how long I will be able to do this," I would tell them, referring to *The Actual Dance*. What surprised me was that, in one way or another, everyone would say to me the same thing: "Sam, write about your MCI. Put it on the page and then on the stage." I did not know how to digest this advice, especially since I was in the middle of the most successful period of booking and performing *The Actual Dance*.

My friends in the New York theater community, mainly members of AND Theatre Company, shared the same inclination. "Write about it, Sam, write about it." For me, it was a whirlwind, almost a tornado of conflicting emotions; I did not know what to do. Then the COVID pandemic hit, and I focused on performing *The Actual Dance* from home. Gabrielle, who was the original dramaturg *for The Actual Dance,* now became my director to create a version of that show that worked over Zoom.

While COVID temporarily ended my touring, it may have also helped hide some of my developing cognitive symptoms. Before the COVID-19 pandemic, as we traveled to theaters and stages in various venues, I had to memorize all my lines. Up until 2020, that was not a problem.

It was during my home performances when I began to need help remembering my lines. At first, it didn't jump out at me as something alarming. It's easy to get distracted performing in a new and confined space, trying to always look at the iPhone camera. More importantly, I had a workaround. Susan was at home, now sitting in a chair just off camera. She was going to join me "on camera" for a discussion with the Zoom audience at the end of the performance. She kept a copy of the script on her lap. I don't remember the first time it happened, just that it did—I needed a cue. I didn't remember the line! She was there to help. I just had to look over to her, and she could mouth the words.

These early flubs hit just as I began noticing other memory issues. Shortly thereafter, I started seeing my doctors, and among my memory complaints included forgetting my lines. The meetings with Dr. Howard, the cognitive testing at the University Hospital Center, and the ultimate diagnosis of Alzheimer's pushed me to the point of trying to write something new. It started in the fall of 2022, and by the end of 2022, I had an idea of what I wanted to write—the story of what by then had happened to me in this neuropsychological world, from oops to MCI and then to the diagnosis in 2022 of early-stage Alzheimer's.

It didn't take me long to draft a short, showcase version of what would become a full play. Yes, writing a 15-minute monologue followed by the full play based on the showcase is a bit nutty. Well, not the traditional way of writing plays.

I kept writing and revising and had a chance in the fall of 2022 to present that 15-minute showcase to an emerging new group named Solo Arts Heal, an informal collaborative of solo-show artists who write on health-related matters. During the COVID years, we partnered with The Marsh, an Oakland, California-based theater. They had also gone virtual. Those of us in the Solo Arts Heal collaborative were presenting pieces—showcases—of our shows as part of a monthly Zoom.

At the same time, I applied to present this yet unfinished play at the Capitol Fringe Festival in Washington, DC, scheduled for summer 2023. I had performed *The Actual Dance* in the 2013 festival, and this was a decade later. The festival itself was recovering from the three-year pause caused by the pandemic, and they were eager for new theatre work. I was immediately accepted, partly because it would be a "world premiere."

All this coincided with the January 2023 APAP (Association of Performing Arts Professionals) conference. It was APAP's return to a post-pandemic, in-person conference and a decade after my first public performance of *The Actual*

Dance. I chose to host a 10th anniversary party, as well as a premiere presentation of a 20-minute preview of the new work, now titled *Dementia Man: An Existential Journey*. Going big, bright, and expensive!

I learned something else during this process in 2023. I began to understand how I was being affected by my Alzheimer's. The symptoms of my growing cognitive decline included significant confusion over planning for and dealing with my big plans. I struggled with the details. I kept calling the APAP staff to get help. I was reasonably well-known among the APAP staff, given my history of attendance. The staff members at APAP were now hearing about my new show, and not just from me. News of a "man on stage with Alzheimer's" was getting some notice. Most importantly, the APAP staff were experiencing and being impacted by my cognitive decline. When I first reached out for assistance about the conference schedules and registration questions, they told me to just "look it up," or read the rules on their conference website. I tried and failed almost every time, so I called them back over and over again, and finally told them about my diagnosis and that I needed their help.

I believe that it was also the first time that the staff of APAP had confronted a person with a cognitive disorder trying to participate fully in the conference. As soon as they had their "aha" moment, they were gracious and fully embraced the succor I needed. I have learned in part from this experience not to give up. My confusion and frequent frustration with navigating what was once ordinary can be accommodated. As it turned out, not only would this first-ever showcase presentation of *Dementia Man: An Existential Journey* be a success, APAP had also arranged for the conference photographer to take pictures of the show, and I was invited to be a guest on the second-year edition of the APAP podcast, called *Arts. Work. Life.*

While I don't know for sure that my show and APAP's introduction to dealing with a cognitively impaired performer were the primary reasons, a year later, in 2024, when I again attended and showcased *Dementia Man*, APAP had added new disability accommodations, including a table for cognitive assistance.

At that January 2023 APAP conference, where I was about to present that first showcase of my yet-unwritten play, *Dementia Man*, I had another problem. One of the reasons I had stopped performing *The Actual Dance* live was that I could no longer remember all my lines. I knew I would not be able to remember my lines for *Dementia Man* either.

For the first time, I had to carry a script in my hands for a performance. It was both necessary and part of the piece's impact. People who experience the show sometimes ask if I "really need" the script in my hand. We have since prepared a sheet for the pre-show introduction stating that holding the script is an accommodation for my disease.

I am nervous on that January 2023 evening in New York City. I have never performed holding the script. I don't know how that will look. The audience is very, very quiet as I perform. I get even more worried. Now that I've been doing theatre for more than a decade, I know that a thousand thoughts can swish through my head in an instant. Then, on stage in the middle of my performance, I wonder, "Why is it so silent? They must hate it." It feels like I am a performer in a vacuum.

I receive my first standing ovation as I finish my last line and bow. I am stunned. As Susan comes on stage to join me, not only does the audience remain standing and applauding, there is also an audible roar.

My next task was to finish the script and develop the direction of the yet-unfinished play. The question of whom to work with on the playwriting was easy for me. Gabrielle Maisels had been the dramaturge for *The Actual* Dance a decade prior and had returned to direct the Zoom version of that show. The big difference was that she no longer lived in the New York area. She and her husband had moved from New York to Santa Fe, New Mexico, where she continues to work in theater and tutors students on the side, primarily via Zoom.

It took Gabrielle and me from January 2023 through the end of May 2023 to finish the script. This involved several public readings and a work-in-progress presentation in New York for friends and family. Gabrielle is always present via Zoom on the iPhone. In the meantime, we needed to find a director. That turned out to be simpler than I thought. A longtime friend and theatrical colleague of Gabrielle's had been directing a theatrical piece in a nearby theatre, just across the Potomac in Maryland, near where we live in McLean, Virginia. In another seemingly impossible coincidence—B'shert, destiny—Gabrielle's friend and our soon-to-be director was living in the Northern Neck of Virginia near where we have a second home. His mother, who had been the director of the regional library there, now Alzheimer's.

The Capitol Fringe Festival had already accepted my play for their first post-COVID festival. The experience of getting ready—the focus on writing, rehearsing—and now getting to walk on stage with early-stage Alzheimer's is to me as complicated an experience as is the disease itself. The symptoms, mishaps, and confusion that can emerge become subsumed by the energy, excitement, and unimaginable graciousness and support of my colleagues and the audiences I encounter. Each performance and almost all since then is met with a thunderous standing ovation.

Typically, every performance is followed by a discussion. Usually, this post-show event is just Susan and me sitting up front, taking questions from—and asking questions of—the audience. Sometimes, there will be a panel of experts with us, like someone from the Alzheimer's Association. There was once a neurologist from the Cleveland Clinic, and another time someone from the NYU Legon Cancer Center who worked on clinical trials.

By late spring of 2023, the word is out. A man with Alzheimer's disease has written a play and is performing it himself! A one-man play performed by a man with Alzheimer's Disease! The bookings come fast and furious, and I perform the play over 50 times by the end of 2024. It is now 2025, and bookings continue, although not quite as frequently. The show evolves, and I evolve. Every performance is unique, and every audience is distinct, and each time, I am inspired by the audience's feedback and appreciation. Once again, I begin learning from my own experiences.

It seems that my engagement with the theatrical world has once again saved me from plunging into depression. It has allowed me to treat the disease as almost a prop. While swimming in the story of my disease, I tend to forget that I do have Alzheimer's disease. It is an odd contradiction for me, and I am playing the role as if I am the actor, not the person with the disease.

Oddly, I did not do what I have done in the past when diagnosed with some medical issues. I didn't run to the Cleveland Clinic or a famous hospital renowned for its work with Alzheimer's for a fourth or fifth opinion. I do know some folks who have done that, even flown to Mexico to try some exotic, unproven medicine in hopes of finding a cure for this incurable disease. I didn't do that. Instead, I wrote about it, and I went on stage.

It also did not take long for Susan and me, as a couple, to come to terms with my diagnosis and settle into the path forward. Yes, we had been here before, so this was not the first time. We'd already had *the conversation*. You know, *The Conversation*, what to do once one of us is diagnosed with a terminal condition.

During Susan's journey with advanced breast cancer, there was a day when the doctors told both of us, Susan and me, that her prognosis was highly guarded. They were faced with the new development of a post-mastectomy lump. Susan and I drove back from the doctor's office in silence, walked into our home, and sat down at our dining room table. I said something to the effect of: "Susan, I am going to take a long leave of absence from my company. We need to take a trip around the world; do all the things we ever wanted to see or do." Susan's response, of course, was: "No, Sam. If we aren't doing what we love or need to do now, then change because of that, not because I might die."

Today, the tables are turned. It is my turn in the terminal diagnosis chair. So, what should I do—should we get in an airplane or on an ocean liner and travel the world? When these questions arise, my symptoms are relatively mild. In addition, I have reached a point in life where, upon reflection, I would be content if this were all there is, even if it all ended today. Indeed, my real job is to figure out how to come to terms with the end of my life.

One option is to accept the end and disappear, literally or figuratively. That might include the suicide option. It might involve, as said by an audience member about her husband, going into my room, closing the door, and not coming out.

I have taken all of these options off the table. No, to a trip around the world. No, to going into my room, curling up, and never coming out. A hard *no* to going to Switzerland.

My answer is different. Yes, and *Dayenu!* An improvised life, lived in gratitude. If the future ended now, so to speak, Dayenu! That is the Jewish phrase from the Passover prayer books used at our Seder, the Passover meal. It means "and it would have been enough." A form of gratitude for gifts from the Eternal for the life I have lived. And today, I do feel Dayenu—if this is all that my life will be, a life that has included a soul partner, two successful and healthy children, and four grandchildren. Dayenu. If this is all there is, it will have been enough. I can't imagine a more beautiful life.

My symptoms are increasing, along with my challenges, indeed, "our challenges." Those are becoming more complicated for everyone in my life circle—my wife, my children, and others around me. At every step, and sometimes daily, I experience new symptoms and "think deeper" about the meaning of this earthly journey, especially in these final years.

Experiencing symptoms, instead of anticipating them, pushes me and moves Susan and me into a new, deeper phase of the disease. It can be scary at times. We are aware of and anticipate the possible radical change in my cognitive situation. It can happen in an instant. I look for an analogy, perhaps as if we are moving from the baby pool to the deep end of the adult pool. Susan is in a little raft next to me, knowing I will sink at some point, and unable to stop it. It isn't as if I step off a curb and get hit by a car. It is when she rolls over in bed one morning and the person there is different than just eight hours earlier. A different Sam.

This journey through my neurocognitive decline will be challenging for everyone. I need more graphic language here. And yet, as I sit here writing this, perhaps even for posterity, I am brought to consider that even in these moments there are gifts. Is the end of life ever happy or good? It is, of course, inevitable. I can't speak to it firsthand, for neither I nor Susan has yet died.

I don't know how other people do it, and I don't want to compare myself to anyone else. Rather, with the gift of having had a fantastic life to this point, with the enormous personal appreciation we—Susan and I—have for our journey together, the things we have been through and have achieved, our family and children and grandchildren and community: the footprints of life we will leave behind, I am back to *Dayenu*. This all would have been enough even if today were my final day.

CHAPTER 12

MY CHANGING REALITY

I am changing. I am living, and I am changing. I have resisted being too explicit about the frustrations and daily challenges in my life. In our lives, Susan and me. There is, though, or so it seems, an opportunity to let the world hear directly from the person with the disease. My entry into this universe of neurocognitive disorders so far has taught me that there are very few voices in this world directly from those who have a neurocognitive disorder. Mostly, we hear from clinicians, partners, caregivers, and various organizations, such as the Alzheimer's Association and various dementia advocacy groups that are emerging in the US.

I love the comments from those who are in the audience after learning about my story. It helps them understand, so they say, what they experienced or are experiencing with a family member with the disease. They tell me that it enables them to make sense of their loved one's bizarre and inexplicable behavior. They can also share the wisdom they have gained on their journey, which is valuable and helpful to Susan and me.

Perhaps some of my ideas and feelings are a conceit. At this point in the journey, I'll take that risk. Some of the experiences you have already read: the disappearance into nothingness. Looking to the right inside my brain, with what seem are tiny eyes sitting inside my brain looking for answers that are not there. I float off instead into infinity. My experience. Delusions are a reality to those of us who have them. Just to be clear, now, at this point, the Nothingness Place delusion, and the scary driving issues have abated. On the other hand, I experience the more traditional symptoms of a neurocognitive disease, such as loss of both short-term and long-term memory and inability to recall words as I speak, though these are just a few examples. While the medications I take have eliminated the delusion of floating off into infinity, the sensory memory of those moments doesn't leave. It is as if The Nothingness Place is just a step away.

Indeed, I sometimes wish there were an experience or hallucination that would at least alert me to my ultimate fall into infinity. The one where I don't come back. I suspect that whatever that moment will be—when I leave—I won't know it has happened. Today, the little slips, and skips, the edge of the abyss, are more frustrating than scary. I keep coming up with the descriptors or phrases. Just the other day, I came up with the phrase *memory clips*. The experience of an idea in my head or thought that just gets clipped and removed. Stolen so-to-speak. I know it was there a second ago, I sorta saw it, and yet it disappeared. Clipped, and stolen.

Susan absorbs these moments and events as they occur because she feels my anxiety and frustration. While not intended for Susan, she can at times become the target of those emotions. We both spend time trying to figure out how to minimize this. Are there words or behaviors we can institute? Maybe the word BUTTERFLY is screamed, and I will know how to stop, breathe, and step back. Or maybe she turns her back. All these assume the cognitive ability to be aware of the moment.

Little and big things. And the advice I get from all those good-intentioned people. "Bring a notebook and take notes." Sure, I would love to do that, except I have dysgraphia by now. I never wrote very legibly anyway—I got an F in handwriting in the 4th grade! Even now, the harder I try, the less legible it is.

I have now developed what I call Groundhog moments, even Groundhog days. Some of the events are funny now, others are just irritating.

One of the first big moments was when Susan and I were invited to a tour of the Kennedy Center. We had been theater subscribers for years, meaning we would purchase a package of five to eight performances a season. We have literally been there hundreds of times before this incident. We had also been members. That meant we paid a fee that entitled us to extra benefits, such as a discount on meals and access to a small member lounge area. Occasionally, we would upgrade our membership level, gaining access to a large member lounge area.

One year, however, we had the good fortune of selling some real estate for a substantial profit, and we needed to take advantage of some tax deductions. We had made a larger-than-usual donation—a higher level of membership. As a thank you, the Kennedy Center invited us to a private tour—well, a semi-private tour—and a private reception with Kennedy Center executives. As our group was escorted in the Kennedy Center Concert Hall, I stopped. Susan was already seated. I remained standing, looking around in amazement. "Wow, it's remodeled!" I exclaimed. "Look at the ceiling, and the side architecture. It's all new!"

Susan stares at me. "What are you talking about? It looks just the same as when we were here three months ago to see Art Garfunkel!"

"What are you talking about?" I respond.

She gently reminds me that we had been to a musical performance by Art Garfunkel three months earlier. I could not pull up an active memory of it at that moment, and while I now accept we were there, the absence of what I call an "active memory" of the event scares the crap out of me.

More recently, I am at home, working on writing this book, sitting at my desk typing away. I get up to stretch and experience an excruciating pain in my left hip. It is as if someone has sliced it with a knife. I nearly fall as I try to avoid placing more weight on my left leg. I had noticed some discomfort over the past few days, although not to this extent. It takes a moment for the pain to abate a bit. I sit back down in my chair and go online to make an appointment with my orthopedist. I type, "New problem, extreme pain in my left hip. Urgent!"

I show up for the appointment a week later, and the nurse takes me into the exam room, opens the electronic screen with my records on it, and turns to me. "You were here six weeks ago for this exact problem, and we treated you." I argue, and so she has me come up to the screen and shows me the image on the screen of that appointment request submitted six weeks before. My earlier request read: "New problem, extreme pain in left hip. Urgent!" None of that triggered a memory. I still don't remember that first appointment, though I believe it happened. Why that event, and not others? I have no idea. It seems so random.

The variations on these experiences are multiplying at an alarming rate. Of course, Susan and I are working on trying to limit the problems. We sit down together several times a week to review the calendar in detail. We discuss upcoming events and deadlines in advance. It helps. It also adds to the complexity of life for both of us, as my impatience with everything grows. I do try to control my agitation, but it is not working well. I quickly seem hostile, angry, and frustrated to her. I tend to raise my voice, mainly because I am frustrated with myself, although to Susan, it feels as if it's aimed at her.

Susan's strengths are vast. She is educated and certified in eldercare from George Mason University. She was Director of Admissions and Marketing at Tall Oaks of Reston, an assisted living facility, for 14 years. She can help people think through their retirement plans and even the placement of their relatives in assisted living or memory care facilities. They were her clients; they leave after a while and appreciate Susan's knowledge and professionalism.

The other difference between Tall Oaks at Reston and now is that she doesn't get to go home, so to speak. In all her work, like the rest of us, perhaps, at the end of the workday, she went home, whether as a teacher for troubled kids or a professional in an assisted living center. Today, in this moment in our lives, it is different. I am reminded of the saying in the legal profession, "A lawyer who represents himself has a client who is a fool."

Today, we are home. She and I are together in ways we never have been before.

Our challenges are accelerating in other ways. I now need Susan or a companion at almost any meeting, especially if something important happens or is said. I need her as I perform my new play, and before I even get on stage. I show up a day early, and we walk through the venue together since I cannot do it by myself. Susan is always with me to help explain things if I get confused, and to occasionally reassure the folks at the venue that everything will be okay.

On the personal side, the other day, I was coughing a lot, and Susan and I became concerned I might develop bronchitis. It was a weekend, and we agreed I should pop into the local Urgent Care. They know me. The doctor asked me simple questions: "When did it begin?" I stumbled and couldn't give a coherent answer because the recent past was already a blur in my head. It didn't matter; ultimately. She listened to my chest, and I got an inhaler and a prescription cough medicine. The cough is going away.

What is lasting, though, is the memory, the frustration, and the realization that I'm entering a new phase of the journey. I shouldn't be by myself in either of these situations.

As I, rather Susan and I, travel these paths through the clouds of end times, we have begun our existential conversations. We are *not* running away from each other or the moment. We do need to make plans, and the tasks are enormous. Just thinking about the mundane of what to do with my vast library—hundreds of precious books. A large house and big questions about whether or not Susan should try to stay here, when it might be time for me to be placed somewhere else. Should we remain here during the closing days of my journey?

There is some good news though. We already have answered the hardest question of all. Our journey together to the end is a gift to each of us—it is, in fact, what love really means. Perhaps because we both have touched the limits, the outer edges of existence; we are uniquely aware of the gifts inherent in being with and holding the person you love as they go through or toward end-of-life moments.

I was blessed to be Susan's love partner through her breast cancer journey. There were times when we both knew or thought we knew that the end was around the next corner. As hard as it was, I found the gifts in that journey. My purpose was to make sure at that last breath, she would leave knowing the infinite love we share, and she would take it with her. As hard as it was, just walking up to that edge with

Susan, I felt it then as a gift to me—a privilege—to be in that liminal moment with her in my arms. These last moments, as we dance around them, are not burdens. They are the pinnacle of what it means to be gifted with the love of another and to create meaningful lives together.

I will not speak for Susan, though we have discussed this. Her journey will be unique. Already, I have been gifted with her touch and soul. I won't have to go to the end to know that, and I don't want to take that opportunity away from her. The complexity is that for her, the body she will hold at that moment, might have become cognitively someone else, someone she never knew and does not know her.

CHAPTER 13

LIVING MY VALUES AS I DIE

While my journey with Alzheimer's isn't always easy for me or my family, that's not what consumes me. I struggle at moments with my need—the irresistible urge from within—to focus my energy during this journey on advocacy for repair and change to meet the urgent needs for reform emerging from the explosion of neurocognitive disorders among the baby boomer generation, and their children.

My goal is to make this last chapter of my life as authentic as possible to who I am and have always been. I worry sometimes if it is unfair to my loved ones. Should I spend more time with my children, grandchildren, cousins, and other family members? My answer has been to listen to my inner voice.

What is an inner voice? How do I explain it? I have always believed in the importance of living my life as authentically as possible. I understand myself as a link in the chain of history of my family. My parents and their parents go back to whatever beginning it was, and then through me to a future that represents them and who we all have been. I do not wish nor believe I should represent a radical departure. I have never felt free to break away from or disclaim the core family traditions or values.

The values that have become ingrained throughout my life now feel integral to who I am. They are not like a book I can put aside or a concert I can leave. This energy, or instinct that lives within me, that forces me to react—to call out injustice—feels molecular, inherent, an "existential" part of who I am as a human being. It is how I have lived my life, raised my children, loved Susan, and caused trouble when what happens in front of me "feels" wrong. Perhaps there is a Myers-Briggs personality type that describes people like me, though I would not mind if I were a new one. Still, I doubt I am unique.

I need to leave this world with those values at play. I want to be a force for change, to be authentic to my core self within the milieu of my life. As I travel along this final journey with Alzheimer's, I am witness to a broken system, a system tied to a history of misunderstanding the nature of cognitive disorders and which heavily discounts the core value of the lives of those with the disease. The social, medical, and cultural infrastructure systems built around us, those with cognitive disorders (major and minor), even today, have failed to keep pace with modernity. The predominant view still discounts the humanity of those going through the progression of cognitive decline. In addition, the social structure we have conflicts with itself. As medicine and medical understanding advance, the myths and fears of the past are promoting strategies for ending lives prematurely.

This is happening as we are approaching a tipping point in the world of neurocognitive disorders. As we see people living longer, physically healthy lives, we are also experiencing a much higher percentage of the aging population living with cognitive disorders.

Unfortunately, there is a growing narrative in society that embraces the idea that the late stages of cognitive decline are unbearable. One book quotes a man with early-stage Alzheimer's as saying: "I don't want to die, but I don't want to keep becoming a lesser and lesser person." The book ends with that person going to Switzerland and committing suicide. The values system behind this movement focuses on the concept of agency, human agency, or the right to die. On one level, this is a debate about ethical philosophy, values, and morals. It is also about "freedom." You, Sam, can do what you want; let me do what I want to do.

I believe in something greater. Societal and social norms create environments that have an impact on existential mindsets or values. When we see something going on around us, repeatedly, it teaches us something. It also creates value systems integral to action. Suicide because of perceived fears of unknowns in the future, I think, should be prohibited. In part, because death is irreversible. One can never change one's mind. I am aware of counterarguments, and I don't want to force-feed people to stay alive. So, I confess here that there are arguments on both sides, and I not only chose life for myself, but I am also willing to live in a society that limits what its citizens may or may not do in terms of killing themselves.

Sadly, one of the major arguments today for assisted suicide is that it costs too much to stay alive with the disease. Patients and their families often face financial challenges, which are frequently unacknowledged, throughout the course of a cognitive disease or disorder, including the final days and the end-of-life period. The challenges argue for public support to ensure that the costs of end-of-life care for those with dementia will not financially destroy a family. It should never be that someone feels obliged to end their life because they can't afford to stay alive.

I believe that people should never be put in a position where their continued life is an unbearable financial burden to their family. Instead, that circumstance should trigger a societal obligation to provide economic support for families whose loved ones need extended care. In what is to me a contradiction, it is the upper classes that seem to be exercising the option to fly to Switzerland, to go through an accompanied suicide. The complaint that I hear, though, is that the person killing themselves doesn't want to "be a burden to the family."

I am pleased to have learned that there are "counter voices" addressing this issue, at least in part by destigmatizing those with the disease and creating narratives of meaning and love throughout the disease journey. It is a growing movement to support and advocate for the inclusion and empowerment of people with cognitive disabilities.

I want to join them to remove barriers and foster norms of radical inclusion of people with cognitive disabilities in everyday society. I also believe that doing so will be of great value to both our social and medical institutions, as well as to the lives of people with the disease. I understand that I am not an expert. It takes a bit of chutzpah to sound off like this right now. I am just another patient, right? What do I know? Well, I think I jumped into the deep end of the pool, and I have figured out how to keep my head above water.

CHAPTER 14

AN AGENDA FOR CHANGE

Fifty years ago, many things we take for granted today, from airbags and kneeling buses to accessible restrooms and assistive technology, were either largely absent or didn't exist at all. We changed the reality then, and we can do it again.

What I hope to do here is to highlight a few of my views on what can and needs to be done now to make a difference in the lives of those of us going through this process. I hope it inspires other changes in the future. At the end of the book, I will also share some voices of experts in the field from which I have found enlightenment and support.

Change The Lexicon, Change the "D" Word

We must change our language around the various forms of cognitive decline and conditions. As previously discussed, at one time, people with cognitive impairments were seen as monsters and freaks. They were called *demented*—mad, crazy, insane. They were put in institutions and kept isolated.

At one time in history, they were viewed as people occupied by demons or even the devil.

We still call that *dementia*, even though the neurological system has renamed the condition, and there is a movement afoot to have Congress pass a law prohibiting the US Government from using that word in materials it creates or funds. Indeed, the word is a modern-day reflection of the history of ignorance surrounding cognitive disorders. Are we still living in Dr. Alzheimer's time when people with cognitive disorders were seen as monsters? Medical and social knowledge had yet to understand what made people change their personalities and lose their ability to function as the same person they had been for most of their lives.

Still, there are more specific diagnoses, and we can see "inside" the brain to find out what is going wrong and often why. I am amused that even in 2025, some people believe that the only way to know if someone has Alzheimer's is in a post-mortem autopsy. While that was true before X-ray, MRI, and PET scans were invented, it is not true today. Interestingly, in 1990, when the Americans with Disabilities Act was initially passed, it did not include cognitive disabilities. It was not until 2008, 18 years later, that it was expanded to include the requirements for accommodation.

Yes, people with physical disabilities have had to fight the same fight—integration into the mainstream of communal living. I saw that firsthand at the World Institute on Disability (WID), as even the most disabled, those with physical, speech, sight, sound, and cognitive disabilities, worked together every day to change the world. And did!

While we know better now, the language hasn't changed much. Terms like *mad, insane, crazy,* and *demented* were the norm to describe the stricken individual. The words *dementia* and *demented* originate from the Latin word *demens,* meaning *out of mind* or *without mind* and are synonymous with *mad* or *insane.* They are not specific to any disease. Rather, terminology is a crude description of how a person with a neurocognitive disorder presents themselves. Or perhaps better said, how people who encounter those with a neurocognitive disorder see or react to them. The word was first used in 1797 for a medical diagnosis and has been in use since the 13th century. The good news is that there is a movement to end the use of "dementia words" in medical and governmental contexts. The goal is to trigger changes in their popular use.

The *Diagnostic and Statistical Manual of Mental Disorders,* 5th Edition (DSM-5) is a manual used to diagnose and classify mental disorders. It's used by mental health professionals in the United States and many other countries. The fifth edition, published in May 2013, replaced the term *dementia* with the phrase *neurocognitive disorder.* It can be categorized as major or minor by the diagnosing physician. The American Psychiatric Association (APA) made this change to reduce the stigma associated with the condition.

The DSM-5 is a standard for language to be used by clinicians, researchers, and public health officials to communicate about mental disorders. In 2013, the DSM-5 also introduced a new category of cognitive difficulty called mild cognitive impairment (or mild neurocognitive disorder). It also replaced the DSM 4 category of delirium, dementia, and amnestic and other cognitive disorders with the "neurocognitive disorders" category.

While it has been twelve years since that change within the medical world, there seems to be little change in the widespread use of the word *dementia*. I observe that this is true in public forums, popular culture, and the medical world, beyond the words written down on insurance forms. The phrase *neurocognitive disorder* does not easily float off the tongue. I have been challenged in this particular issue—what to call what I have—because of the title of my play, *Dementia Man: An Existential Journey*, and I am sure now this book. "If you hate this word so much, why do you call your play *Dementia Man*?"

Yes, the contradiction defines the problem. I hope to be part of that change, and plan to transition from *Dementia Man: An Existential Journey* to *An Existential Journey: My Alzheimer's Story*. That should work for me. I hope, too, that I can help normalize "cognitive impairment" or "cognitive disorder" as everyday language or phrases.

We have a model for this language change. There is another word, much like the word dementia, which was in popular use for a very long time. This word dates back to 1426 and has become commonly referred to as the "R" word. It is derived from the word "Retarded."

"Retarded" was previously used as a medical term. The verb "to retard" means to delay or hold back, and so "retard" became known as a medical term in the late 19th and early 20th centuries to describe children with intellectual disabilities or *retarded mental development*. Up until around the 1960s, the terms "moron," "idiot," "cretin," and "imbecile" were all genuine, non-offensive terms to refer to people with mental intellectual disabilities and low intelligence. These words were discontinued in that form when concerns arose that they had developed negative meanings, with "retard" and "retarded" replacing them. After that, the terms "handicapped" (United States) and "disabled" (United Kingdom) replaced "retard" and "retarded". *Disabled* is now considered a more polite term than *handicapped* in the United States as well.

On October 5, 2010, President Obama signed S. 2781 into law. Known as Rosa's Law, the bill changed references in federal law; the term mental retardation was replaced by mental disability. Additionally, the phrase "mentally retarded individual" was replaced with "an individual with an intellectual disability." Rosa's Law was named after Rosa Marcellino, a nine-year-old girl with Down's syndrome. She worked with her parents to have the words "mentally retarded" officially removed from the health and education code in Maryland, her home state. With this new law, "mental retardation" and "mentally retarded" no longer exist in federal health or education and labor policy. The rights of individuals with disabilities would have remained the same. The goal of this word removal was to eliminate language that may be perceived as hurtful by individuals with the disease and their families.

In 2025, a new advocacy movement was launched called the Initiative to Change the "D-WORD." (https://

notdemented.com/mission) The founder and leader, Mike T. Zuendel, graciously participated in an interview for the *Dementia Man* webcast. He is attempting to use the model of Rosa's Law. Now, we need to stop using the term *dementia* in any federally supported program, document, or initiative. Maybe we will name it Mike's Law!

Access to Support: Cognitive Navigators for All!

I sometimes wonder how or why I got so involved in the disability movement in the United States. As I have written already, I was on the board of directors of the World Institute on Disability for 15 years. I was privileged to meet and get to know some of the early icons of the American disability rights and advocacy movement. At the time, I had no known disability. I had a touch of dysgraphia—well, just terrible handwriting, cursive or printed. I was punished in grade school for my terrible handwriting as if it were simply a matter of will. In the fourth grade—and yes, now, 70-some years later, I still remember and picture my time in the classroom, after school, alone, with the teacher who had me spend a full hour writing letters in cursive on the blackboard, over and over again. In retrospect, I think it was a disability, especially since it has only gotten worse over time. I finally found accommodation. I became a speed typist. In law school, I would type my homework and exams if I felt confident. If I didn't, I would handwrite them. I am convinced that the teachers would give me the benefit of the doubt if they couldn't read my handwriting because I spoke well in class, and they believed I knew my stuff.

I get distracted; yes. I was writing about the World Institute on Disability. It was founded in 1983 by Judy Heumann, Joan Leon, and Ed Roberts. I got to know them all, though I didn't join the board until about 1995. Deborah Kaplan, who had worked for my company, Issue Dynamics, Inc., became the executive director of WID. I served as a board member for about 15 years, developing relationships and learning from many of their staff and other board members. Most notably, for the purpose of this book, I saw in real time how significantly disabled people lived meaningful, productive lives with their disabilities.

As I reflect on why I believe and want to engage in the world today, now with Alzheimer's, just as I did before, or perhaps better said, "as a normal, aging 80-year-old," I attribute the reason in significant part to my experience of having deep engagement with WID and other disability advocates years ago. I have seen and experienced in my own life that differently abled people can engage and add value to our community every day and in every way. It is possible! Often all it takes are small adjustments in how we design our architecture or systems to welcome and accommodate everyone.

Indeed, it is the time I spent and the engagement with so many people with advanced disabilities that enables me today to imagine that I, too—and others with neurocognitive disorders—can live an engaged, meaningful, and productive life, with accommodations, for a significant period, even with this disease, even as I get worse.

What did it take to enable people who needed help walking or were in wheelchairs? Elevators and ramps, and enough taxis that use cars with room to store wheelchairs. What does it take to enable blind people to travel? Taxis, Ubers, Lyft, etc. Or theatre or operas for the blind? There is now audio description. Give the blind person a device for them to hear a person describe the stage action as it happens. Buses and subway systems have braille signage and safety strips on the ground. Those who are deaf can read, and real-time electronic captioning is often the most important accommodation.

These are all things we take for granted today. What we don't see, though, at least not yet, are systems for those of us who get confused or don't understand even some of the simplest directions. How do we enable mild to moderately cognitively impaired people to travel and engage with our communities? Let me give you a recent example of the challenges we encounter doing routine "things."

The other day, I drove to a nearby restaurant in Bethesda, Maryland to have lunch with some friends. There was a city parking lot right across the street, with an open parking spot near the main entrance. I pull into the spot and see a sign: "1. Note your parking space number. 2. Buy your ticket for up to two hours. 3. Go." They even have a note at the bottom: "Simple."

I walk to the machine and stare at it for a few minutes. I cannot figure out how to activate or start it. I don't quite understand the "theory" of the new parking system. As I stare at the machine, a woman, seeming around my age, approaches to use the machine next to me and does it effortlessly. I ask for help, and she tries to explain what I need to do. She stands by as I fumble through it, then points out that I had been successful because my ticket is sitting in a small slot at the bottom of the machine. When I open it, I see that I have purchased two tickets. I have paid twice. At least I didn't get a parking ticket for not paying.

I acknowledge that this task of redesigning our public-facing systems to accommodate those of us with neurocognitive disorders is challenging. A simple answer, which I reject, is that it is my or my family's responsibility always to have a companion. Which reminds me, we do allow dogs as companions on everything from trains to planes and buses. Even pets for emotional support, as well as guide dogs. Typically, we don't charge extra for them. If I need a human being to help me, I have to pay double.

Most people can't imagine a world with a much broader availability of support for people with cognitive decline than we have now. It is partly because we rarely see cognitively impaired folks, except in institutional settings. In part because the word "dementia" evokes late stages of the process, when for many, the journey from beginning to late stage can last years, even decades. This "late stage" bias is ingrained in our institutional systems and our minds, and it needs to be changed. A public consciousness of the challenge ahead is possible, as possible as it has been accommodating physical disabilities. New systems that will ultimately prove to be helpful to everyone must come "online" in almost every public-serving place that exists.

Here are just a few ways to achieve that goal. The first and foremost is the concept of cognitive navigator and cognitive navigation —people and service agents trained to work with or even alongside people with cognitive impairments, and systems designed to include those with cognitive impairment in daily life activities. Implementing these solutions can be simple or complicated, as you will read.

Retail: Cognitive-Friendly Stores

For those with physical disabilities, there are ramps into every store, cuts on every curb, special desks, and checkout stations with lower (wheelchair high) counters. There is braille signage in elevators, as well as audio announcements for the visually impaired and signage for the deaf.

There is almost nothing for those with cognitive disorders, though there are emerging changes in some locations.

For those with cognitive issues, there could be more frequent, larger, and clearer signs outside the elevator with bigger or simpler lettering, listing the tenants and their locations. There could be more help desks, and potentially, real smart, AI functioning devices with "NEED HELP? ASK HERE."

Now, imagine every Walmart and Target and local grocery store having carts with a sign on the front that says: "I have cognitive disability," and a counter or location with a big sunflower sign, with a staff person trained in cognitive navigation support. A check-out line with the Yellow Flower signs for checking out with assistance. Yes, there could be cognitive navigators—trained people—to walk with customers who need help throughout the store. One day, that might be a robot, also AI-powered, that can be given your shopping lists, read shelf signs, and may even know the "best deals" available.

Recently, with the increased delivery services by many stores, especially grocery stores, I have noticed employees filling electronic orders. They could also be available to escort those of us with cognitive disorders as we shop. Why not?

Similarly, websites could be designed for greater cognitive accessibility, allowing those with cognitive challenges to engage online without feeling overloaded and overwhelmed.

Neurological Medical Services

As described in this book and my play, today's patient is typically confronted with a badly broken neurological medical system. These issues may be common around other terminal illnesses.

In the neurological world, from where I sit, the challenges start when a person or their loved one experiences concerns and symptoms and reaches out for help. It continues through diagnosis, treatment options, and life's final days. Yes, I have some insight into the parts of the journey I have gone through and in which I am now living. My views expressed here on the later stages are more tentative. I am not there yet and don't expect to have the capacity to write much once I enter late-stage disease. I smile as I write this last sentence.

It isn't clear to me why the neurological infrastructure struggles to deliver treatments, care, and information for the patient world. I understand that, in part, this is due to the lack of positive medical therapies and the absence of cures. I know, for example, that Alzheimer's disease is the sixth leading cause of death and the only one without any cure. There are many other diseases that are primarily neurological or have associated effects, such as Parkinson's.

There is one thing that can be done right now, which would have major impacts on the medical experience. Every medical practice or office of a practitioner should be required to provide cognitive navigator assistance and support in their medical offices. This could be required by redefining the standard of care needed by medical associations or by insurance companies. I am not trained well enough to specify the details of that support beyond talking about what would have helped Susan and me: a trained social worker who would have sat down with us to offer information about resources in the community, along with an explanation of the likely path forward, and to whom we could ask questions. Instead, we swam in a sea of uncertainty and confusion for months. Yes, these services must also be covered by insurance and Medicare.

Planes and Trains

In the United States today, many airports offer lanyards with green and yellow flowers for individuals with cognitive disabilities to wear around their necks. It identifies them as someone who needs help. So far, I haven't seen those in train or bus stations, though we clearly should have them.

I imagine cognitive-navigator-type support for those who need guidance or even someone to walk them onto the train, plane, or bus. Maybe even stay with them to their destination. Right now, if you want someone to be assigned to get you where you are going, typically you have to get a wheelchair. That is at least door-to-door. There are electric carts, too, though they don't have a high level of one-on-one assistance. There is growing training of airport staff about what the lanyard means. Susan and I recently experienced that at an airport while going through the TSA checkpoint, wearing my lanyard. After I put my luggage on the moving belt and started to walk, alone, toward the x-ray scanner, the agent helping asked Susan, "Are you with him?" He had noticed my lanyard. She said yes, and he told her to move ahead and that he would take care of her luggage. All that is great, and perhaps there could be "disability lanes" staffed by individuals who could provide specific trained support for those requiring extra time, and simpler language, whether for movement or cognitively. This might free up the other lines to move faster.

In train stations, at least on the East Coast, assistance is left to the porters. Airports didn't develop with this type of history, though airport porters are also available. At train stations, getting to your train, the right car, and seat is more complex, so having cognitive navigators to help—along with specific signage or a desk (or desks) for that type of support—is necessary. Perhaps the same green and yellow flower design—make it universal—will help. The compensation systems, with which I am not that familiar, will also need to be changed so that the cognitive navigator doesn't have to rely on tips, and the person who needs help doesn't have to pay for that type of help.

I have spent many years as an inter-city commuter. There was the time I had an office for my company in San Francisco, and I traveled from the DC area to California once a month. I did that for about seven years, and once found myself in medical urgency. I had developed a blood clot in my leg and have ever since had to watch for thrombosis in my legs and lungs. So having wheelchairs and attendants was helpful. Later in life, I was commuting from the DC area to New York City every other week. I knew the train stations and could get into the elite lounges where they had Red Caps meet us and help. I don't travel so often now, so I don't get private lounge privileges, but I do go routinely to the Red Cap area. I have imagined a cognitive navigator—think super Red Cap (Amtrak's free baggage handling service)—who I could arrange to meet me at the front door of the train station after being dropped off by my wife or a cab, who would be my cognitive navigator until I am on the train and in my seat.

Whether the train or the plane, I want the attendant to be trained to recognize those of us who need extra time and deeper explanations and know how to best engage us. Now, there are other transportation modes, such as cabs, car services, and Greyhound buses. I imagine they, too, should have their staff—drivers—trained for our needs. I realize that slightly different solutions might be required for each type of transportation; trains are different than planes. Uber and Lyft use contractors, not employees. I believe solutions will emerge once the requirements are defined and implemented. In part, because the number of "clients" with these impairments is going to grow dramatically, and there is money to be made from serving us.

CHAPTER 15

LAST WORDS

There is a narrative that asserts that life for those with progressive cognitive disorders is not worth living. There is a similar narrative for our life partners, husbands, wives, and perhaps even children. "I didn't sign up for this!" Though I have not heard it, I worry that my kids and grandkids might be thinking this.

Wouldn't it be better, then, to just develop some easy exit ramps for those who don't want to drive this route? We've been on a superhighway most of our lives. Now, we have to go up and down these treacherous mountain curves. Hell, I was about halfway through an intersection the other day when I remembered I needed to turn right, which I did anyway (not good). Then I forgot the appointment was at 1 p.m. and nearly missed it. Thank goodness I got a call to ask where I was.

Is this the end I bargained for?

How long do I have to live? I can tell my cognitive capacities are declining, and I don't always have control of my emotions. You have read the story to this point in my life. I do not want to go, to disappear, or to die. Yes, I'm still me, the 80-year-old version of that. Yes, I have all sorts of things happening to me, and like every other human being ever born, I will die.

Where does my desire to live a meaningful life for me, my family, and the larger communities of which I am a part of come from? As weird as it sounds, that desire feels inherent, or genetic. An existential part of "me."

Every human being is distinct; the assemblage of genes and lived experiences molds us into a unique human being.

I believe that every day I take a breath, even the day I change to become someone else, I will always be a troublemaker—the one who always sees a way for something to be fairer or better.

I believe that no matter what happens in the coming years, I will be the best of whatever I am that the world has ever seen. In some ways, it is a truism because I am the only one of me that there is. It feels like we are going in circles, doesn't it? And yes, to a degree I am.

In this moment, let me give credit to my friend, the late Lynn Fielder, who taught me that our mission in life is to be the best we can be of what we are and have been given. Lynn passed away at 62 from her Parkinson's disease, diagnosed when she was 30. She taught me the life lesson of embracing ourselves as we are, not as we wish we might have been, and that we must do that as fully, graciously, and meaningfully as possible. Lynn, by living her life with that disease so fully and generously, gifted many of us—her family, her daughter, and me, at least—a perspective on living with grace and meaning until the very end. Thank you, Lynn.

I want to acknowledge how hard that can be. Every circumstance is different. I do see, in particular, the complexity of living with this disease and the financial impact on a family. If my health care ended up draining every penny of our resources and then bankrupting our children (if they would do that), would my last five to ten years have been worth it? Is that logical? Is that moral? Because our—Susan and my—circumstances are such that such an outcome is not within our sights; I don't have to live in that moment, and I do not want to judge it. Instead, I hope we can envision a larger community in which individuals in such circumstances are provided with dignified care and support as reasonably needed. Yes, this language is a bit of a cheat. I know the goal is challenging. I repeat: it is not a morally acceptable system to have people ending their natural lives because they can't afford the care.

My imagination is for a graceful end, with existential love, no matter what happens. I get to speak from experience. Indeed, Susan and I have both walked through the valley of the shadow ... Each is now experienced as a patient and a caregiver. We have come to understand that there is no greater act of love than being the partner of another. In that process, we experienced a form of grace that transcends words. It is existential, knowing and experiencing the nexus or connection with another, both in the existential moments of living and dying.

I once was at a conference where each attendee had to be a "presenter," as well as an audience member. I was on a stage at a session where our responsibility was to offer "last words"—whatever that phrase meant to us. Five minutes. It was improvised in real time in front of a group of highly accomplished individuals. In those moments, I discovered something that has changed me and allowed me to navigate my existential journey, however it ends, with confidence and love, not fear. The last words I said would be:

> *I am sorry ... for anything I have done to hurt you.*
>
> *I forgive you ... for anything you fear you may have done that hurt me.*
>
> *I love you ... for you are the other half of my whole—my existential partner in this lifetime of wonder.*

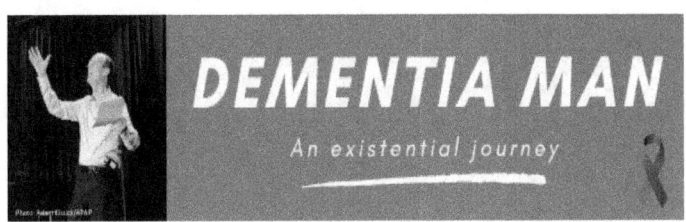

DEMENTIA MAN POETRY

GOING AWAY

It never occurred to me that I am going away.

Invited into our neurologist's private office for this visit.
We sense that something must be wrong.

The neurologist does not look up. He seems reserved.
"Early-stage Alzheimer's disease," he mumbles.

It never occurred to me that I am going away.

I now wonder what it will be like.
It has its own allure.
Will the present Sam simply evaporate?
Is it a place of great peace?
Maybe the pain is just in getting there.

Yes, I am going away. I wonder what it will be like.
A new place of the present only.
No memory of me now.
Every day a brand-new start.

I wonder: What will the Sam of me then, know of the Sam of me now?

I am not afraid, just curious.

THE FUTURE FADES

Why is it that I can see with great clarity moments in my history while visions of a future fade?

Moments remembered:

The grid metal of a floor furnace in our home
 Imprinted as a scar on my right calf when I was 2
The giant leap off the ledge of our front porch when I was 5
 Transformed to a small step down for a grown man
Staring up from the floor, at the radio blaring, *The Lone Ranger*
 It became a waist-high piece of furniture much later
The morning of the day Grandpa died; I was only 4
 The cries in the halls as my parents wept
10-year-old me slapping mud on my face in the backyard
 Aunt Julia picks me up and tells me to stop
The moment in a room, saying goodbye
 To a sister whose mind worked differently

Moments unseen:

The agenda for today, much less for tomorrow.

Our Anniversary Day – now approaching 60 years.

Where I am going, for just a moment, waiting for the light to turn green.

And of course, where I put my keys and my glasses.

IN BETWEEN NOW

I am in between now.

Vague recollections of what has been, forgetting what just happened.

In between now.

Was it really me?
Was I there?
Why did I get that invitation?
How do I do that? It used to be so simple!
What used to be so clear is now a maybe.
The past is fading more rapidly.

In between now.

There will be a time soon when everything will be new.
Even me.
In between can be a dangerous place.
Arguments and denials, only vague recollections.
Sensing the frustration and hurt in others.
Trips and falls. Getting lost in my house.
Perhaps it will be better when I reach the other end.
The new me—with no knowledge of the past.
Every moment a surprise. No struggle to recall.

Getting through the in-between, to the other end, can become, at times a tempting thing.

NO-THING-NESS

A play on life – or is it death – or maybe just words.
Except it is real – this no-thing-ness place.
It has no light, no sound,
No smell, no feel, no taste.

No beginning and no ending.
And, thankfully, no other people.
At first, I thought it was death.
Then I come back.

No-thing-ness is a dilemma.
For me it is real.
By definition, it is not.
If it is nothing, then it is not anything.

Yet I know when I am not.
The moments that feel like years
Then back again
In and out, lost and found, dead and alive.

I savor the moments when I can still pretend.
I write a poem and perform an entire play.
I am fine, then slip away and return. Again.

There will be one time, I know.
Yes, just one. It will come.
When I slip away into that no-thing-ness.
And stay.

US

Life exists within each of us as a form of the Divine.

A tangible essence of who we are.

Love is when our essence became entwined.

Each an equal half of the other.

"I love you" simply awakens the **US** in you and me.

From Sam to Susan

APPENDIX

WORDS OF CAUTION

The journey with a neurocognitive disorder typically starts before we know we are on the journey. The symptoms aren't always apparent. It is different for everyone. My experience, as described in this book, spans nearly a decade.

I struggled with changes I did not recognize as a disease or a disorder. I was just bothered by them, and my doctors minimized them. First, it was suggested that they stemmed just from stress; then the underlying cause became "normal aging." This is not unusual, I have learned, and during these early periods, we can easily fall for schemes or quick-fix medicines. Many of these, often supplements advertised on television, are marketed with the claim that they will keep us sharper.

Fraud and misleading information have been and continue to be a personal challenge for many of us. There are so many promotions and advertisements for "cures" and "secrets for better results" that it is frightening, even for me. At first, I would see them on television, usually cable stations, and now they are on digital platforms like Facebook. Or worse, my internist once gave me a book with a title suggesting it provided a way to "end Alzheimer's," and we just needed to spend $10,000 to visit a spa treatment center for a week.

Please, dear reader, if you or anyone you know feels their memory or cognition has changed, first consult a medical professional. Standard testing is available that can measure your cognitive abilities against a population just like you. A primary physician can do some of it, though a neuropsychologist or neurologist would be best. In many areas of the country, there are hospitals with memory clinics and practices.

Even then, a neurocognitive disorder can be challenging. On my journey, I have heard many stories that aligned with my own experience of a doctor discounting a patient's concerns. Often expressed with the same words spoken to me. *Normal aging.* Or. *It's not that bad.* Or. *It's just stress.* Here is a tip if this happens to you. If your doctor is telling you not to worry about something that is bothering you, or seems to be discounting it, ask a straightforward question: *"Okay, and what else could it be?"*

If you are still not satisfied, look for a second opinion. Find a specialist, usually a neurologist. You can ask for a referral from your primary care doctor. If that is uncomfortable or impossible, sometimes you can make an appointment on your own, without a referral, and be seen. There are memory centers within many major hospitals. They are often interested in finding people at the early stages for possible drug trials. I have in the past sought a second opinion from the Cleveland Clinic in Cleveland. (They have affiliations and branches in other cities.) While insurance won't pay for transportation costs should you have to travel to a different city, like me, so far my insurance has paid the medical bills for second opinions.

A second opinion once saved me from having a very invasive surgery. It turns out that I had been unlucky enough to have one of these "rare side effects" from a routine "minor procedure." One way to resolve that "side effect" was a brand-new surgery, and the doctor to whom I had been referred pushed me hard to have the operation. The Cleveland Clinic doctor, one of the leaders in this field, handled the immediate issue simply and non-invasively, and said, "Get another local doctor."

I know this journey can be tough, and I offer these words of caution in hopes that if you find yourself with concerns about your memory, you will look for quality medical support. I also note that even in that world, care and vigilance is required. Another option is to find a trusted friend or neighbor who has been through the process or has a family member with the disease.

Even though I was a high-performing, high-profile professional, I struggled greatly during the time I began to experience symptoms and sought out a diagnosis. I have since discovered that there are several government-based resources—as well as some patient-based organizations—I wish I had known about. Here is a list of some of those resources:

GOVERNMENTAL RESOURCES:

The ADEAR Center

The Alzheimer's and related Dementias Education and Referral Center (ADEAR) provides evidence-based information to people living with Alzheimer's and related dementias and their families, health care professionals, and the general public. They provide answers to specific questions about Alzheimer's and related dementias. They have an 800 number, which I have used, and it was helpful and reliable. They offer free articles and publications about dementia symptoms, diagnosis, related disorders, risk factors, treatment, caregiving tips, home safety tips, and research. You can contact them at 800-438-4380 (English & Spanish, 8:30 a.m.–5:00 p.m. ET, Monday–Friday). Or email them: adear@nia.nih.gov

Alzheimers.gov

Alzheimers.gov provides information on Alzheimer's and related dementias, a searchable database of clinical trials, and resources from across the federal government. In addition, the Alzheimers.gov Virtual Assistant offers a quick and easy way to find information about Alzheimer's and related dementias. They provide information on disease and ongoing clinical trials, and links to other federal support resources. They have a newsletter, too, that I have found reliable and helpful. The National Institute on Aging, including its ADEAR staff, also manages the Alzheimers.gov website. They share the contact information: Phone: 800-438-4380 (English & Spanish, 8:30 a.m.–5:00 p.m. ET, Monday–Friday) Email: adear@nia.nih.gov

NON-PROFIT AND PATIENT-BASED RESOURCES:

ALZHEIMER'S® ASSOCIATION

The Alzheimer's Association is a leading voluntary health organization dedicated to Alzheimer's care, support, and research. Its mission is to eliminate Alzheimer's disease through the advancement of research, to provide and enhance care and support for all affected, and to reduce the risk of dementia through the promotion of brain health. The Association offers a wide range of services, including a 24/7 Helpline (800-272-3900) for information and crisis assistance. It also provides personalized care consultations, online resources such as ALZConnected®, and tools for legal, financial, and care planning. The Alzheimer's Association advocates for public policies that increase funding for research and improve access to quality care. https://www.alz.org

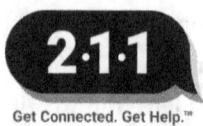

A national non-profit platform that exists in every state and community, the 211 phone and online program will connect you to government-based resources, both local and federal, in any state. You can start at the national or state level. For example, https://211virginia.org/ takes you to a menu of statewide government resources. Most importantly, these are going to be reliable, credible, and vetted. Each menu contains resources for "aging & disability" as well as many other conditions. www.211.org

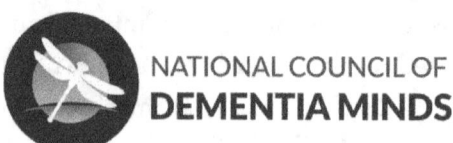

Insights of Persons Living Well with Neurocognitive Disorders

National Council of Dementia Minds identifies itself as the first national 501(c)(3) organization founded and governed by people living with dementia. They include individuals with all types of dementia or mild cognitive impairment, including younger-onset dementias. Their mission is to develop and support a national corps of Dementia Minds groups—composed of people living with dementia—that foster education and dialogue among individuals with neurocognitive disorders, families, care partners, healthcare providers, researchers, and policymakers. https://dementiaminds.org/

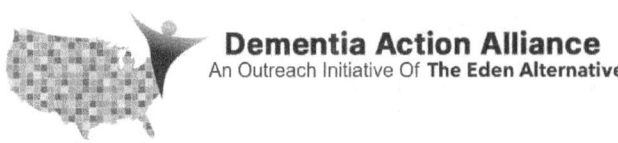

Dementia Action Alliance
An Outreach Initiative Of **The Eden Alternative**

Dementia Action Alliance

The Dementia Action Alliance, DAA, describes itself as a diverse coalition of passionate people creating a better society in which to live with dementia. In 2025, Dementia Action Alliance became an outreach initiative of The Eden Alternative, Inc., which the IRS recognizes as a charitable 501(c)(3) nonprofit organization. DAA was founded in 1996 as a national advocacy and education organization of people living with dementia, care partners, dementia specialists, and other advocates, and remains functioning in this capacity within The Eden Alternative. https://daanow.org/

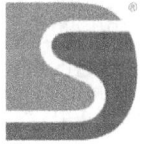

Dementia Society of America®

Dementia Society of America® (DSA) is an all-volunteer organization that addresses all forms of dementia. It has an information request hotline (1-800-DEMENTIA®), to help locate many online resources. It also underwrites nonmedical activities through its Ginny Gives® Program, which focuses on music and singing, dance and movement, the visual arts, touch, and sensory stimulation. https://www.dementiasociety.org/

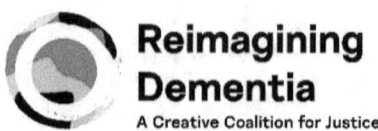
Reimagining Dementia
A Creative Coalition for Justice

An initiative led by Reimagining Dementia: A Creative Coalition for Justice, Taking It to the Streets calls on its 1,100-plus members and many other allies to host public-facing events, activities, and conversations that present a creative alternative to the fear, stigma and hopelessness surrounding dementia. https://www.reimaginingdementia.com/takingstreets

East Side Institute

The Joy of Dementia (You Gotta Be Kidding!)© is an experiential workshop hosted at the East Side Institute which uses improvisational games, creative exercises, and philosophical/performed conversation to create an environment that supports everyone involved in the "dementia ensemble" to transform the "tragedy narrative" and creative environments that support possibility, growth, and hope. https://eastsideinstitute.org/the-joy-of-dementia/

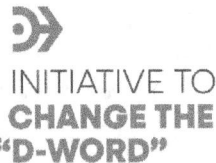

INITIATIVE TO CHANGE THE "D-WORD"

The Initiative to Change the "D-Word," is an organization founded by Mike T. Zuendel, a business entrepreneur who was diagnosed with Alzheimer's disease. After treatment with a new drug to reduce his amyloids to normal levels, he was inspired to start a movement to eliminate the word "dementia," which he finds degrading. He considers it as intolerable as the word "retarded." His goal is to convince Congress to eliminate the use of the word in federal medical work and thus trigger a larger change. Since 2013, the neurology medical materials have begun using the term "neurocognitive disorder" rather than dementia. https://notdemented.com

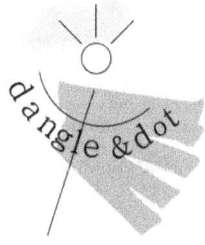

After Nancy (dangle) was diagnosed with Alzheimer's, her friend, Kat (dot), became her care partner. They are amazing advocates and have organized themselves into a program and resource for others going through this journey. They are big fans of *Dementia Man*. They described their work as an

effort to help others imagine "doing dementia differently." This is how they put it: *We, with our energetic enthusiasm, optimism, and lifetime of experience, want to empower you to dare to do dementia differently, and live life well, with purpose, for longer.* www.dangledot.com

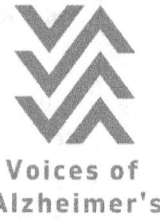

Voices of Alzheimer's

The Voices of Alzheimer's is a national advocacy organization devoted to, as they say: *Empowering people living with or at risk of Alzheimer's and other cognitive illnesses, united by urgency, to drive equitable access to innovation in treatment and care.* The organization, a 501(c)(4) not-for-profit advocacy initiative, engages in political advocacy on behalf of its members. https://www.voicesofad.com/ There is a partner non-profit foundation that focuses on educational activities and donations to them. Unlike donations to The Voices of Alzheimer's, those to the VOA-Foundation are tax-deductible. https://www.voa-foundation.org

APPRECIATION

MY MOST IMMEDIATE FAMILY

Susan M. Simon (Cognitive Navigator – LovePartner™):
It feels awkward giving Susan a place here when, in fact, her contribution to my life and this journey is incalculable. Not only is my wife of 59 years taking this journey with me, she has also become my caregiver. My love and appreciation for her are best expressed in my prior book *The Actual Dance: Love's Ultimate Journey Through Breast Cancer*. She is the other half of my whole. She is my model of how to focus on seeking to be the outlier, the unlikely survivor.

Susan holds a master's degree in special education from George Washington University and has served as an elementary school teacher. She also served as an elementary school counselor. Susan then received a certification in eldercare from George Mason University. She served as the Director of Admissions and Marketing at Tall Oaks of Reston, an assisted living community, for 14 years. We have two adult children and four grandchildren. Susan has served on the boards of the Fairfax Education Association and the Jewish Council on Aging and is a past President of Temple Rodef Shalom, Falls Church, Virginia..

Children and Grandchildren:

I haven't included them before in my "thank you" sections of books and the like. I felt compelled to acknowledge them on this, my anticipated last book and play, for no other reason than how fortunate Susan and I are, and how proud we are. In reality, there is no assurance that families—children and grandchildren—will be loving, successful people committed to each other and historic family traditions and values. Ours are, and we value and appreciate that. I can't imagine this journey, especially now, if we were traveling amidst disruption and dysfunction. We feel extraordinarily blessed. Just a shout-out to them for being them:

Marcus and Rachel Simon

Marcus is our firstborn, and Rachel is his wife. They live in Falls Church, Virginia, only 10 minutes from our home. Marcus is a lawyer and an elected official. He is a senior member of the Virginia House of Delegates, representing the 13th District. His wife, Rachel, works for a charity—Tickets for Kids—that persuades major arts and sports venues to donate tickets to children. They have two children: Emily, who just graduated from the University of Delaware, and will be finishing a master's degree next year. Zachary just completed his freshman year in college at Virginia Tech and is entering his sophomore year.

Rachael Simon and David Proper

Rachel is our second-born, and David is her husband. She has chosen to retain her maiden name, primarily for professional reasons. She is a pediatric dentist, so technically, she is Dr. Rachael Simon, DDS, and lives with her husband, David Proper in Marriottsville, Maryland. So, they are either 45 minutes away or three hours in traffic. David Proper has worked part-time and served as a part-time stay-at-home dad. He is now working in the family business and supports the administrative needs of the dental practice. They have two daughters. Sydney finished high school this year and is planning to attend Widener University in Pennsylvania, on a lacrosse scholarship. She is an outstanding athlete. Joanna, her younger sister, is a junior in high school, very active in the B'nai Brith Youth movement, and herself a strong athlete, having served as captain of a volleyball team, and is currently running track for her high school.

DEMENETIA MAN, AN EXISTENTIAL JOURNEY – THE PLAY

The Creative Team:
Gabrielle Maisels (Dramaturg & Co-Director)

Gabrielle Maisels has served as the Dramaturg to the playwright and was an essential collaborator in the development of the show. She has also served as my acting coach. She is an actor, playwright, and acting coach, and the writer/performer of two solo shows, *Two Girls* and *Bongani*, inspired by her family's experiences in South Africa. Gabrielle studied political theory at Harvard and Columbia, acting with Carol Fox Prescott, and playwriting with Matt Hoverman. New York theatre includes: Solo shows in Fringe NYC 2010 and 2011, Clear Cold Place by Caroline Prugh, Agnes in Tony Kushner's A Bright Room Called Day, Esther in Kushner's Terminating, Rocky in Men of Clay (Off-Broadway, with Matthew Arkin, Danton Stone, Steven Rattazzi). Member Actor's Equity. www.gabriellemaisels.com

Thadd McQuade (Director)

Thadd McQuade has been a director, teacher, and performer for 40 years, splitting his time between classical and Greek theater and new experimental works. He has worked internationally with the Odin Teatret and Teatr Gardzienice and has produced multiple shows at the Edinburgh Festival Fringe. His work there has been nominated for a Total Theatre Innovation award and won a BBC Most Innovative on the Fringe award. For the last four years, Thadd has been working on ways to expand the work of theater to incorporate neuro-diverse voices and artists.

THE BOOK

Coach:

Linden Gross (lindengross.com). So how do you write a book of a story that I wrote as a play? You would think that a guy who had three books under his belt, including a book picked up by Book-of-the-Month Club as a premium gift when that was a thing, would know how to do this. Well, not so much. I pat myself on the back for finding Linden Gross, whose supportive and innovative style has helped me transform the play into an actual story in this book. Her patience, support, and discipline adapted to my crazy style have gotten me to the finish line and across.

Readers:

I benefited from a few talented experts and writers who graciously reviewed the text and provided feedback. They have become friends and colleagues in this journey as well. Please don't blame them for anything in the book, I didn't take all their suggestions, just most of them.

Harvey Freedenberg

Harvey Freedenberg has been writing about books since 2005, and in that time has published more than 1,250 reviews, essays, interviews, and columns. A member of the National Book Critics Circle, he has written for print publications and websites that include BookPage, Bookreporter, Shelf Awareness, Kirkus Reviews, and the Minneapolis Star Tribune, as well as several literary blogs.

Harvey is a retired lawyer. He concentrated on the fields of intellectual property law and litigation.

Mary Fridley

Mary Fridley is on the faculty at the East Side Institute in NYC, co-creator and leader of The Joy of Dementia (You Gotta Be Kidding!), and coordinator of Reimagining

Dementia: A Creative Coalition for Justice. A long-time community builder and developmentalist, Mary practiced social therapy for 12 years and uses the social therapeutic approach as a teacher and workshop leader. She is the author of several articles and chapters on the Joy of Dementia and the Coalition. Additionally, Mary is a guest blogger for *agebuzz* and a playwright and theater director.

Steve Gurney

Steve Gurney is a nationally recognized leader, innovator, and advocate in the field of aging and longevity. As the founder of the **Positive Aging Community** and **Positive Aging SourceBook**, Steve has dedicated over 35 years to empowering individuals, families, and organizations to make informed decisions about aging and senior living. Inspired by his family's experience caring for his grandfather, Steve launched Retirement Living SourceBook (https://www.retirementlivingsourcebook.com) in 1990, creating a comprehensive resource that quickly expanded across the Mid-Atlantic to serve the DC metro, Maryland, and Philadelphia regions.

Steve has served on the boards of numerous aging sector organizations, including the **Alzheimer's Association**, **Interages**, and the **Beacon Institute**. He has been recognized with awards from **Seabury Resources for Aging**, **Southern Gerontological Society**, **Insight Memory Care**, the **Aging Life Care Association**, and other notable organizations. A frequent speaker at local, regional, and national events, Steve is regularly featured in media and has served as an adjunct professor at the **Erickson School of Aging Studies at UMBC**, instructing at both undergraduate and graduate levels.

Rev. Lynn Casteel Harper

Lynn Casteel Harper is an essayist, minister, and chaplain. Her debut book, *On Vanishing: Mortality, Dementia, and What It Means to Disappear* (Catapult, 2020), was named a *New York Times Book Review* Editors' Choice and a Chautauqua Literary and Scientific Circle selection for 2021. *Vanishing* appeared on the Gold Foundation's 2021 Reading List for Compassionate Clinicians.

A graduate of Wake Forest University Divinity School and Robert Wood Johnson University Hospital's chaplain residency program, Lynn has served as the Minister of Older Adults at The Riverside Church in the City of New York and as a nursing home chaplain. An ordained Baptist minister (Alliance of Baptists), Lynn lives and writes in Bridgeport, Connecticut, where she is the pastor of Olivet Congregational Church UCC.

Frances W. Schwartz

Frances Weinman Schwartz is a writer and educator specializing in Jewish subjects. She has lectured extensively and is a facilitator for a course in Wise Aging at her synagogue, Temple Micah, in Washington, DC. Currently, Francie serves as a senior editor at *Moment* magazine. Francie received her master's degree in Judaic studies from Hebrew Union College and is a graduate of the Medill School of Journalism at

Northwestern University. Prior to turning to Jewish studies, Frances was a journalist working at television stations in Chicago and later worked on documentaries in New York. Frances is the co-author of *The Jewish Moral Virtues* and *A Touch of the Sacred*, books she wrote with the late rabbi and eminent liberal Jewish theologian Dr. Eugene Borowitz. Francie is also the author of another book, *Passage to Pesach*.

Frances lives in Potomac, Maryland, just outside Washington, with her husband, Stuart. She's the proud mother of Dana and David, and three grandchildren, Jonah, Teo, and Stella.

SUPPORTERS OF *DEMENTIA MAN*
(as of publication--for a current list see: www.dementiman.com/donate)

Co-Executive Producer
Susan M. Simon

Associate Producers
Dr. Rachael & David Proper * Christian & Judy White * Rabbi David Saperstein

Contributing Producers
Elisa Joseph Anders * Bob & Blythe Chase * Daniel Davis & Karen Menichelli * Evelyn & Eugene Fox * Patrick Gaston * Rick & Susan Gorsky * Pamela Hagan * Mitzie Hiegel & Larry McAlistor * Lee Hougen * Nancy Kane * Sue Pickens Owens * Stephanie Pelmoter * Margery Rosenberg * Bertrand Schreibstein * Dr. Jay Sanders * Charlie Shafer * Rachel & Marcus Simon * Mavis Springer

Assistant Producers
Helen Able * Malcom Avner * Grant & Margaret Bagley * Julianne Brienza * Teddy Burris * Linda Davidson * Lisa & Seth Feder * Barri & Kirby Fogel * Jonathan Ginsberg * Judy Gray * Marilyn Herman * The Keppler Family * Gail Kropf * Jeffrey Lepon * David Lord * Sidney Louick * Andrew Joskow & Lisa Sockett * Lisa Mackem * Mark McFeely * Allen Leider * Beulah Levy * Karen Pyeatt * Joanna & Kenny Raskin * Carol Saferstein * Sandra Saydah * Howard Smith & Beth Singer * Gregg & Monty Skall * A Lynn Snow * Jody Wager * Robert Wu * Melanie & Scott Zucker

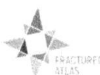 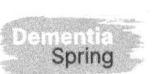 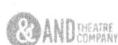

ABOUT THE AUTHOR

Samuel A. Simon was born in El Paso, Texas, in July of 1945. He was raised in El Paso and graduated from the University of Texas at El Paso in 1963. He was married to Susan Kalmans on August 23, 1966, in Houston, and they celebrated their 59th anniversary in 2025.

Dementia Man: An Existential Journey is the second play created and produced by The Actual Dance, LLC. It made its world premiere at Capital Fringe in Washington, DC, in July 2023.

Sam Simon was diagnosed in 2018 with Mild Cognitive Impairment and in 2021 with Early-Stage Alzheimer's. He is currently under medical treatment and a participant in a drug trial.

He has brought together his experience with his first play, *The Actual Dance: Love's Ultimate Journey Through Breast Cancer*, which serves as a vehicle to reach those going through the disease, his history as a leader in the American Disability Community, and his new life experience engaged with dementia to develop what he hopes will be a dramatic statement on the possibility of productive life after such a diagnosis.

Sam Simon describes himself as being engaged in his fourth-age of life, as a playwright and performer. He likes to say that this period of his life found him. Although Sam is a seasoned writer and author, he's an unlikely playwright and performer. He started as a lawyer committed to America's consumer movement. He was an original participant in Ralph Nader's first legal advocacy group, The Public Interest Research Group, in 1970. He and his work have been featured in national media, including *The New York Times, The Washington Post, Face the Nation, Good Morning America, Today, The Phil Donahue Show, The Oprah Winfrey Show,* and other outlets. He is the author of three books and the editor and compiler of another.

In the late 1990s, Sam was introduced to and trained in theatrical improv at Artistic New Directions, now AND Theatre Company in New York. He became a member of Gary Austin's Workshop in New York and Washington, DC.

His first play, *The Actual Dance: Love's Ultimate Journey,* debuted in 2013 and inspired a memoir by the same name published in 2012. *Dementia Man: An Existential Journey* debuted in 2023, in the Capitol Fringe in Washington, DC. Since then, the play has been performed throughout the United States. Information about *The Actual Dance: Love's Ultimate Journey Through Breast Cancer* is available at www.theactualdance.com, and information related to *Dementia Man* is available at www.dementiaman.com. Sam also invites readers to connect with him directly at sam@dementiaman.com.

www.ingramcontent.com/pod-product-compliance
Lightning Source LLC
Chambersburg PA
CBHW071234070526
44583CB00017B/2174

So, What's Grief Really Like?

a book about grief and loss

Susan-Rose McIntyre